The HANDBOOK OF HOMOEOPATHY

A comprehensive introduction to the subject of homoeopathy for
both practitioners and all those interested in a deeper
understanding of this system of medicine.

THE LOGIC OF HOMOEOPATHY

The HANDBOOK OF HOMOEOPATHY

Its Principles and Practice

Gerhard Koehler

Translated from the German by
A. R. MEUSS F.I.L., M.T.G.

THORSONS PUBLISHING GROUP
Wellingborough, Northamptonshire

Rochester, Vermont

First published in the United Kingdom 1986
Second Impression 1987

First published in West Germany as *Lehrbuch der Homöopathie*
© Hippokrates Verlag GmbH, Stuttgart 1983

© THORSONS PUBLISHING GROUP 1986

British Library Cataloguing in Publication Data

Koehler, Gerhard
    The handbook of homoeopathy: its principles
    and practice.
    1. Homoeopathy
    I. Title   II. Lehrbuch der Homöopathie.
    English
    615.5'32   RX71

    ISBN 0-7225-0992-8

Printed and bound in Great Britain

CONTENTS

Preface to the Second Edition

The first edition of this book found its buyers within a very short time, a sign that there is a lively interest in homoeopathy.

It is always possible to improve on a book, but no changes have been made for the second edition in order to avoid an extended period out of print.

I should like to express my gratitude to all the people who have had a hand in the making of this book.

Freiburg im Breisgau, FRG
January 1983

G. *Koehler*

Preface to the Fourth Edition

The first edition of this book appeared in 1982. Three years later I am delighted, grateful and full of hope in writing this preface to the fourth edition.

I should like to express my gratitude to the many readers of this work and to the publishers. Delight has come with the realization that the homoeopathic approach to medicine is gaining new friends. And there is hope that in the dialogue between the different schools of medicine discussions are getting more unbiased and objective as we face our common task — to achieve a gentle and lasting cure for our patients.

Freiburg
In the spring of 1985   G. *Koehler*

PREFACE

The medical profession of today ought to consider themselves fortunate, for their diagnostic and therapeutic armamentarium very likely holds a greater potential than ever before.

Scientific analysis has given useful results for many areas of medicine, and the technical perfection of the apparatus used in diagnosis and emergency treatment is very high indeed. Surgery and prosthetics are now able to help beyond the limits set in the past. Depth psychology offers insights into dimensions of the soul that were formerly unknown. Psychosomatic medicine is beginning to reveal the interaction which exists at many levels between body and soul.

We may well call ourselves fortunate as we contemplate all the advances made. Yet in the daily work with our patients we very often find ourselves in crisis situations. Why is the number of chronic cases on the increase? Is it really only due to civilization and an increased life expectancy? Why are we so often forced to weigh the benefits of a potential treatment against the harm it may cause? How are doctors and patients to evaluate the risks and contra-indications of a particular drug when the manufacturers themselves are not fully aware of them, the reason being that it often takes a long time before they are in evidence? On the one hand we are having to face the dangers threatening our environment and on the other we also see with deep concern the threat to the inner world of man. We find ourselves exposed to harmful agents present in the air, in the water we use and the food we eat, and also to the harmful effects of drugs.

The 'crisis situation in medicine' which we have been hearing of for the last fifty years is undermining the confidence of both doctors and patients. A solution can only be found by first of all looking for the root causes of the crisis, so that we may take united action. The German author Peter Bamm identified these root causes as follows:

The scientific basis of medicine is experimental biology. It is known, however, that experimental biology does not in fact concern itself with the study of life, but rather the analysis of the physicochemical systems on which life is based. Medical therapy based exclusively on experimental biology can only address itself to abnormalities in the sphere of life that are abnormalities in those physicochemical systems. A physician will not find this adequate in dealing with his patients.

The metaphysical uneasiness which has been a groundswell in medicine for a whole generation arises because being what it is, the scientific basis of modern medicine cannot encompass the situation a medical practitioner faces at the bedside. The physician has to deal with a patient whose medical disorder includes disorder in the transcendence of the patient's person. . . .

Medicine will have to include the whole sphere of life and its entelechial regulation if it is to have any prospect of not only restoring biological functions to normal but to heal the sick person. (*Ex Ovo*)

I am deliberately quoting from a neutral source, for the idea of a crisis situation in medicine has not been generated within homoeopathy. A sufficient number of people in orthodox medicine today are sensitive to the unease which prevails and are looking for new ways. The situation is challenging all of us to look for more comprehensive approaches to treatment.

Homoeopathy has much to contribute to medicine as a whole. It has proved itself both safe and effective over a period of 180 years. Above all it treats the sick individual as an integral unity of body and soul, seeing him as someone playing an active part in life who is partly determined by his individual constitution and human environment and subject to the conditions and stresses of his period and biography. The sick person as an individual and an integrated unity of body, soul and spirit sets the standard in homoeopathic medicine.

Different therapeutic approaches within the whole field of medicine have their strengths and their weaknesses, depending on the individual situation.

It is time therefore to stop being arrogant and contentious and instead opt for brotherly co-operation. All of us owe a duty only to the patient, not to any ideology or particular therapeutic approach. We can all learn from each other.

I feel greatly indebted to those who taught me at medical school and to my clinical training. Yet it would be wrong for any of us to stand still at the point reached on graduation.

'We have reason to rethink our medicine. The advances made in medical science, the desperate situation in the field of medical training, the problematical structures of health services and increasing problems of making medical practice meaningful are the subject of highly critical attention. Our efforts in dealing with health, sickness and suffering, with need, debility, helplessness and crisis situations, are influenced by the tension which exists between the potentials for medical action and the limits to such action.'[1]

Anyone who has come up against those limits in his daily work with patients feels challenged to look for other potential methods of healing. Professionally, and indeed legally, we are in fact obliged to do so.

Rising above conflicting views and methods we can use the words of Samuel Hahnemann, the founder of homoeopathy, as a touchstone for the quality of our work and our aims in medicine:

The highest ideal in medicine is the rapid, gentle and lasting restoration of health or the relief and eradication of the disease in its entirety, choosing the shortest, most reliable and least detrimental route, our reasons for the choice being clearly perceptible.

Many of the older generation of physicians, but above all also young doctors and medical students have come to realize that it will be possible to overcome the therapeutic crisis which is one of the crises in medicine by giving serious consideration to natural methods of healing. Increasing numbers are attending postgraduate courses in homoeopathic medicine. Medical students in particular are asking for training. Unfortunately medical schools are still resisting those demands, though time is getting short, with many patients abandoning the doctor's surgery for a visit to a lay practitioner — a phenomenon which ought to be taken very seriously in professional politics and medical schools.

This book has developed out of a seminar for homoeopathic medicine which developed in response to requests from the student body at Freiburg University Medical School.

To provide additional material for the students I produced scripts every semester (half year) and these gradually formed a whole volume. At the insistence of my students I then decided to rewrite this material which had proved such an effective teaching aid and make it into a book. It is hoped that it will contribute to and encourage further dialogue between the different approaches used in medicine.

I am greatly indebted to all who have helped to make this book a reality — the publishers, especially Mrs B. Huwald, their reader, and Mr Klotz as managing director; Mrs Ilse Laessig of Freiburg who has been most helpful and brought her lively intelligence to the work of typing the manuscript; and last but not least my colleagues and students who considerably influenced the work through stimulating collaboration and criticism in the courses and seminars.

Freiburg im Breisgau, FRG
July 1981   G. *Koehler*

---

[1] Seidler, Woerterbuch medizinischer Grundbegriffe p. 13.

The Position of Homoeopathy within Medicine

Anything we do to help sick individuals may be said to fall into one of three categories. We are able to reduce the strain on the patient's functions, to support those functions or to exercise them.

Depending on the individual case, the one or the other of these categories will be appropriate.

A patient with a fresh myocardial infarction must first of all be put on strict bedrest and the strain on cardiac function reduced. After this, coronary and myocardial function are supported. Finally, rehabilitation is the aim, with a suitable exercise programme.

Reducing the strain and giving support to functions usually calls for nursing care and medical treatment. Physiotherapy uses natural stimuli such as light, air, water and movement to improve the patient's ability to function through exercise.

Providing exercise means to apply a stimulus. The organism improves its autoregulation by reacting to this. Most of the methods used in orthodox medicine today have the emphasis on reducing the strain and supporting functions or else they serve to suppress undesirable reactions. A point to be considered is whether the increase in morbidity particularly as regards chronic diseases may not be partly due to this.

With any stimulus used therapeutically it has to be remembered that it is not the power of the stimulus but the power of the reaction which determines the result.

The sweeping statement 'the bigger the better' obviously does not apply with any form of exercise therapy.

Rehabilitation after a heart attack starts with minimum exercise loads. Oertel's treatment for example starts with very short walks, cautiously increasing the distance whilst monitoring the reaction, so that a training effect is just discernible.

The traditional Kneipp method uses minimal stimulation with cold water applications to part of the body that will just cause a slight reddening and increase in skin temperature. Unfortunately the tendency today is to use anything but subtle stimulation. Pastor Kneipp poured the water from a can the size of a medium-sized watering can for indoor plants (on exhibition at the Kneipp Museum in Bad Wörishofen, FRG). A full bath was a 'horse cure' in his eyes and only used in very exceptional cases.

In his principal work, *The Organon of Practical Medicine*,[1] Hahnemann recommended the application of cold water if there was a lack of vital warmth. He may be considered to have been ahead of Kneipp in this respect.

It is interesting to note that Hahnemann put his finger on the seeming paradox of any form of stimulant therapy: cold applications to treat lack of warmth.

There are no objective standards for the strength of stimulus to be applied. It is the reaction which determines it, and this brings in a completely new standard: the subject himself. It is the reaction produced by the subject which determines the measure and degree of stimulus. Physical stimuli generally have an alternative effect on the autonomic system and hence on capillary tone. They are nonspecific, with no primary effect on specific organs or tissues.

Medicinal agents are much more specific. 'There is remedy for everything', the saying goes, but the question is which remedy for which disease and which particular patient? In the past, healers found the answer to that question through generations of empirical observation and near-natural instincts.

Experiments as a method of putting specific questions to nature have had their precursors in antiquity and during the Middle Ages, but it was Francis Bacon (1561-1626) who gave them their present significance as a major element in scientific discovery.

Bacon's principal work was called the *Organon*, and it is surely not by chance that Hahnemann, too, called his principal work an *Organon*. His life work started with an experiment.

Hahnemann asked himself the specific question: What reaction does a drug produce in healthy human subjects?

He was not satisfied with speculative explanations such as that a drug acted as a 'stomachic', that it had nutrient, derivative, liquefactive or alternative properties. His answer was clear:

A drug produces an artificial disease. Like any other foreign material it provides a specific stimulus. Its only curative effect lies in eliciting a reaction from the organism.

His type of experiment, consisting in drug trials on healthy subjects, demonstrates that drug actions meet the criteria for the category of stimulant therapy:

1 Every drug provides a specific stimulus and this is characteristic of that particular drug.
2 The stimulus has to be accurately defined to achieve a useful reaction.
3 The reaction depends on the initial state of the organism.
4 Small stimuli have a stimulant effect due to a reactive response from the organism. More powerful stimuli force a direct primary effect. Massive stimuli are toxic.
5 It is the subject who determines the appropriateness of a stimulus by the nature of his response.

The last point demonstrates the difference in therapeutic approach between allopathy and homoeopathy. To achieve a laxative effect with aloes, a powerful dose is 'appropriate', having a direct stimulant effect on the gut. If the gut is already irritated, e.g. in a case of colitis, a minimum dose of aloes will be 'appropriate'. The artificial disease induced by aloes is a state of irritation. If such a state is already present as an authentic disease, subtle doses of aloes may relieve the condition. A substance is able to cure the conditions it is able to induce. It absolutely depends on the initial state. The authentic disease and the specific artificial disease must show similarity.

The difference between the two approaches emerges clearly if we define their areas of application.

Homoeopathic medication does not replace missing substances; it does not aim to compensate a component system by the direct route; it does not counteract reactive processes and suppress them. Homoeopathic medication has a regulative effect on the central controlling processes in the organism.

Every living organism follows an inherent law of life in constantly endeavouring to remain in balance. The maintenance of balance depends on adaptive reaction to internal and external stimuli. The response to stimulus depends on the initial state of the organism; its aim is to achieve a 'steady state' (von Berthalanffy), i.e. homoeostasis of vital functions. The ability to respond to stimulus is what distinguishes the living from the dead. The ability to maintain a steady state is what distinguishes normal from disease states.

Factors interfering with the internal balance will trigger regulatory processes such as pyrexia, inflammation, vegetative alteration (Hoff).

Some of these regulatory processes, pyrexia for example, are apt to take the form of quite vehement reactions. Interpreted as necessary

The Handbook of Homoeopathy

Table 1

Principle of medicinal action		Examples
Substitution	Replace missing substances	Iron deficiency anaemia Insulin for diabetes
Compensation	Balance defective systems	Digitalis glycosides in congestive cardiac failure Diuretics in nephrogenous oedema
Suppression	Reduce undesirable or excessive reactions	Cortisone for allergic reactions Betablockers for premature beats Antibiotics (sulphonamides, penicillin) for infections
Regulation	Control pathological processes	Desensitization using minimal doses of allergens Immunostimulation, e.g. tuberculin vaccine Homoeopathy

regulation applied by the 'inner physician', they become a 'healing illness.' The indiscriminate use of antipyretics may interfere with the process of immunoregulation. Suppression prevents the body from regulating itself. Past generations of physicians have often been better observers. Celsus, a Roman physician, felt able to say: 'Give me a drug that will produce a fever and I'll cure every illness.'

If the organism's own regulative reactions are excessive or inadequate, medical art will have to assist the 'inner physician.'

'Assist' does not mean suppression, however, nor short-term overstimulation or autoregulatory mechanisms. The aim of homoeopathic treatment is to stimulate the autoregulatory system to heal itself and to control it in a meaningful way. It helps the body to help itself. *Natura sanat.*

It is only possible to control the autoregulatory mechanisms if the initial state of the individual patient is taken into account. This initial state may be recognized from the reactions shown by the individual, i.e. the symptomatology. Objective signs and subjective symptoms serve as pointers to where abnormal reactions are occurring in the individual case.

The objective clinical findings make it possible to give a name to the disease, to classify the disorder. The subjective symptoms go further than this, providing insight at a deeper level, so that the sick person may be grasped as a unique individual.

The individual has to be seen as unique. This one particular individual has to be seen by the physician as a whole consisting of body, soul and spirit.

The regulatory processes we have so far been considering more at the physiological level assume deeper significance at the individual personal level. Disease consists in a disruption of the central regulating energies that maintain life. Hahnemann called this central principle the 'immaterial life force, dynamis or autocracy', Aristotle referred to 'entelechy', others to the 'life principle'. These are different terms for something man finds it impossible to put a name to. Yet each of us knows that we are living out of those 'depths', out of a sphere science cannot reach. This is the sphere of things that cannot be measured or weighed and are not open to experimental proof.

Psychosomatic medicine and all forms of psychotherapy are working at this level, using the word, dialogue, as their tool. In so far as due consideration is given to the subjective element, all psychological disciplines have something in common with homoeopathy.

In the weighable and measurable sphere of the physical body modern orthodox medicine has many points of contact with homoeopathic medication. The definition of homoeopathy as a particular form of regulatory therapy will help to establish mutual understanding.

As a school of medicine which specifically considers the individual person, homoeopathy endeavours to integrate the disciplines concerned with the treatment of the soul with those concerned with the treatment of the body. That is no empty phrase. The testing, selection and action of a homoeopathic drug always covers the symptoms and signs in body, soul and spirit, and these are always considered as a totality.

[1] Frequently translated as *Organon of the Art of Healing*. Translator.

2

THE PRINCIPLES OF HOMOEOPATHY:
HAHNEMANN'S LIFE WORK

Within the total context of medicine, homoeopathy may be defined as a specific form of regulatory therapy.

The founder of homoeopathy was Samuel Hahnemann. His method of practical medical treatment is based on three principles:

Drugs are tested on healthy human subjects	The whole clinical picture is considered on an individual basis

Law of Similars,
matching symptoms obtained in drug tests
against the individual clinical picture

1 Definition
Within the total context of medicine, homoeopathy may be defined as a form of regulatory therapy. The aim is to influence autoregulation with the aid of a drug which relates to the way the individual patient reacts.

2 Founder of Homoeopathy
The founder of homoeopathy was the German physician Samuel Hahnemann (born 10 April 1755 in Meissen on the Elbe, died in Paris on 2 July 1843).[1]

He became a member of the medical profession at a time when there were two opposing trends in the field of medicine — on the one hand 'Romantic Medicine' (Leibbrand), intellectually brilliant but also speculative, on the other hand the practitioner at his 'trade', using very radical therapeutic methods. Excessive bloodletting, clysters and other derivative measures (fontanels) weakened patients for no apparent benefit. Medical treatment consisted in heroic doses of mixtures containing many different drugs. The actions of these had never been tested experimentally nor determined empirically. Instead of experience and scientific analysis there was speculation, and blind faith in authority meant that spurious knowledge had been passed on from generation to generation ever since Galen's day, a method on which Paracelsus in his day had poured scorn.

Hahnemann was born in Saxony, a country improverished by the Seven Years' War (1756-63). His father was a porcelain painter, not a lucrative trade. Samuel Hahnemann was highly gifted as a linguist and as a student earned his tuition fees and living expenses by doing translations. He was proficient in Greek, Latin, English, French, Hebrew and Arabic. His work as a translator provided him with deep insights into the medical, pharmacological and chemical literature of his day. He added his own critical comments and annotations, his chosen motto being *Aude sapere* — 'Be bold and be sensible' or, more freely translated, 'Have the courage to think for yourself.'

Independent thinking made it necessary to contradict the authorities. Translating Cullen's *Materia Medica* he came on a speculative statement by the author to the effect that Peruvian bark (*Cinchona* species, homoeopathic name *China*) cured intermittent fever because it acted as a stomachic. This statement set his critical mind aflame.

3 Drugs Tested on Healthy Human Subjects

In 1790 Hahnemann started to investigate the claims made by Cullen and with the sublime certainty of a genius tested the drug on himself to determine its actions. That was the moment homoeopathy was born. Its first principle was established experimentally: The actions of a drug are determined by testing it on healthy subjects. Testing Peruvian bark on himself he experienced changes in his subjective state of health that resembled the symptoms of intermittent fever. He wrote:

> As an experiment, I took about four drams of good quality *China* twice daily for a number of days. First my feet, fingertips etc. grew cold and I became languid and drowsy. Then I developed palpitations, my pulse grew hard and rapid, intolerable anxiety, tremor (but no shivering) and enervation in all limbs. Then a pulse was beating in my head, redness of cheeks, thirst — in short all the symptoms familiar to me as belonging to intermittent fever made their appearance one after the other, though there were no actual attacks of chills and fever. In short, the highly characteristic symptoms of intermittent fever I am familiar with — dullness of the senses, a kind of stiffness in all joints, and above all the unpleasant sensation of numbness which seemed to be located in the periosteum of all the bones in my body — all made their appearance. The paroxysms

always lasted for 2 or 3 hours, recurring only when I repeated the dose. I stopped taking the drug and I was well again.[2]

4 Law of Similars

Hahnemann formulated this, the second of his principles, in 1796. He published a paper entitled 'An Experiment Concerning a New Principle for Determining the Medicinal Powers of Drugs' in *Hufelands Journal*. His 'new principle' was the testing of drugs on healthy human subjects. His brilliant conclusion reads as follows:

> Every active principle provokes its own kind of disease, as it were, in the human organism. We should imitate nature, for she often cures a chronic disease with another which comes in new. When it is a question of curing a particular disease (especially chronic disease), we should therefore use a drug which is capable of provoking another, artificial, disease that resembles the original disease as closely as possible. *Similia similibus.*[3]

To stress the point, let me repeat part of that conclusion: '. . . capable of provoking another, artificial, disease'. Drug tests on healthy subjects initiate an artificial disease and the symptoms of this should as closely as possible resemble those of the disease we are treating. Drug action resulting in man-made disease is something we are all too familiar with today since the introduction of chemical drugs. In a somewhat shamefaced effort to play things down such man-made diseases are referred to as 'side effects'. It is a definite understatement to describe the devastating results seen in some patients as 'side effects'. Remember Hahnemann's motto *Aude sapere* — Have the courage to think for yourself.

The Law of Similars, first put down in print in 1796, was given its final classic form in Hahnemann's *Organon of Practical Medicine*:

To achieve a gentle, rapid, certain and lasting cure, always choose a drug capable of provoking a disease similar (*homoion pathos*) to the one it is to cure. (*Organon of Practical Medicine*, Introduction).

The Latin phrase *Similia similibus curentur* puts it succinctly (Let likes be cured by likes). The Law of Similars bases on comparison between the total pictures presented by two sets of facts. The patient's symptoms are matched against symptoms produced by the action of the drug in healthy subjects, making a phenomenological comparison.

5 Individual Disease Picture

The name given to a disease — the diagnosis — refers to the registration of pathological data. This is dependent on the current state of knowledge and subject to constant change. For the practical application of the

Law of Similars it is however necessary, for obvious reasons, to consider the individual symptoms of the patient and not a collective disease concept.

Comparison can only be made between elements that are comparable. The symptoms a patient presents with can only be compared with the symptoms produced in drug tests.

Hahnemann's *Organon* gives exact directions as to how a history should be taken to elicit the individual disease picture and which symptoms determine the choice of drug in the individual cases (§§ 83-104).

Summary

Homoeopathy is a form of medical therapy based on regulatory principles. It stimulates and controls autoregulation. Samuel Hahnemann, the founder of homoeopathy, developed a system of medical practice based on three principles:
— Drugs tested on healthy human subjects
— Law of Similars
— Individual disease picture.

The Law of Similars calls for likes to be cured by likes (*Similia similibus curentur*). The comparable 'simile' is to be found from among the characteristic symptoms produced in drug tests on the one hand and the symptoms individual to the patient on the other. Comparison of these two sets of symptoms leads to selection of the drug showing the greatest similarity in the individual case. This drug is therefore referred to as the 'simile'.

---

[1] For further literature on the life of Hahnemann see Index of Literature: Haehl, Richard; Tischner, Rudolf — historically accurate. Fritsche, Herbert — the cultural and intellectual background to homoeopathy is brought to life. Ritter, Hans — a highly critical review; the genial aspect of Hahnemann's work fades beside the image of a man living in a particular age.

[2] From Cullen, *Abhandlung über die Materia Medica*. Band II, p. 103 ff.

[3] *Hufelands Journal* 1976; II:434. English translation in *Lesser Writings*.

3
THE DRUG

Homoeopathy endeavours to obtain accurate knowledge of drug actions from four sources:
— Drug tests on healthy human subjects
— Data from toxicology and pharmacology
— Clinical use
— Use and experimental studies in animals.

The totality of these data is known as the 'drug picture'.

The drugs used in homoeopathy derive almost exclusively from the kingdoms of nature (plant, animal, mineral), and only a few from synthetic compounds.

Hahnemann used a specific technique (trituration or succussion) for the processing of raw materials. The raw materials are step by step taken to high attenuations. This allows their qualities to unfold and enhances their efficacy.

Hahnemann therefore called drugs prepared by this method potencies or dynamizations.

The *Homoeopathic Pharmacopoeia* gives definitive directions as to the processing of homoeopathic drugs.

It is crucial to know as much as possible about drug actions on as comprehensive a basis as is possible considering the present state of knowledge. Action in this case means — and this cannot be sufficiently stressed — the changes a drug produces in body, soul and spirit. Drug action means that an (artificial) illness or disease is produced. Anything caused by a particular agent can also be cured by that agent. It is this which makes it a medicinal agent. 'Anything which causes illness also has medicinal virtues.'[1] Every drug has two faces, being both medicine and poison. Knowledge of drug actions is obtained from the study of drug-induced diseases.

1 Sources of Drugs Data

DRUG TESTS ON HEALTHY HUMAN SUBJECTS

It is not possible to elicit the specific medicinal actions of a substance by *a priori* methods — speculation or deep thought, intuition or correspondence based on the *signatura rerum*.

Hahnemann ranks among the first scientists to use experiments in order to put specific questions to nature.

> This type of pharmacology should exclude all assumptions, unfounded statements, and above all, all that is invention. Let the language be that of nature in response to careful, honest questioning. (*Organon*, § 144)

The oldest path to knowledge, one that has always proved its value, is by observation and experience. Experimentation substantiates observation and experience and adds new observations. Lets us hark back once more to Hahnemann's Peruvian bark experiment. There had been definite, repeated experience that *China* was effective in certain cases of intermittent fever. It needed an experiment, however, testing the drug on himself, to show Hahnemann why and when *China* would as a rule be helpful. In healthy subjects *China* will produce changes that resemble the syndrome experienced with intermittent fever.

Doubts have been expressed as to any real value of drug tests on healthy subjects.

> Statistical analysis of repeat tests done by P. Martini showed them to have been inconclusive, the trial method having been inappropriate. The group of subjects must cover a wide age range and both sexes. Tests with *Sepia*, a drug used particularly to treat menopausal women, were predominantly done on young subjects. The only older female subject (no. 8, aged 53) produced a beautiful *Sepia* symptom: 'remarkably indifferent to anything unpleasant, things that would normally upset her'. A sensitive musician (no. 6, male, aged 39) reacted by being weepy and sad, with restless sleep and general nervousness.
>
> Martini made an interesting comment: 'On the other hand a particularly striking feature was that in both test series the relative frequency of symptoms tended to be less when low potencies and the mother tincture were used than with the higher potencies (up to 10x)'.
>
> Statistical analysis ignores the few rare and peculiar symptoms that are of qualitative significance.

The realistic value of such tests can be shown with examples taken from everyday life. I am sure you have all wept copiously when peeling or slicing an onion, with your nose itching until you have to sneeze. The irritant effect an onion has on the eyes and nose is common experience. It is also well known from experience that many catarrhal conditions produce similar irritation of the eyes and nose.

Do you remember your first attempt at smoking, maybe resulting in your dirtying your pants? Remember how you felt dizzy, had to hold on to something and felt dreadfully sick? You had turned a pale green. Do you remember the effects of tobacco? I am sure you have also seen patients who — for quite different reasons — felt so dreadfully sick and giddy that their face showed a deathly pallor or looked green and they had to hold on to things and go and lie down. That is the appearance of someone in a state of circulatory collapse. Attacks of this kind often occur with Ménière's syndrome.

Do you like coffee? Perhaps there has been an occasion when after some time without you had a cup of really strong coffee. Soon you felt really 'wound up', there was a rush of blood to the head, your heart beats grew rapid and hard. At night you found it impossible to go to sleep, new ideas kept coming into your head and you were tossing and turning. Surely you have heard similar symptoms described by patients (often women approaching the menopause).

These have been examples to show — at least in rough outline — the reality of drug action as you all know it from experience. You have been 'testing' *Allium cepa*, the onion — *Tabacum nicotiana*, the tobacco plant — *Coffee tosta*, roasted coffee. Latin names instantly make quite everyday things appear more scientific. Everyday things become scientific when data are collected on the basis of experiments. Data are gathered in systematic tests with medicinal agents.

Hahnemann tested drugs first on himself, then on his family. He got friends, patients and colleagues to take part in the tests and later, when he taught at university, also some of his students. Initially the drug under investigation was given in measurable quantities, in a single dose, and Hahnemann asked for detailed accounts of all subjective symptoms and objective signs noted by the subject. If there had been no change, the dose would be increased a few days later, and he would continue to increase the dose until there was a definite reaction. Hahnemann's directions as to how these drug tests were to be conducted were exact and extremely precise for those days (*Organon*, §§ 105-8, 120-53). He was the first to carry out drug trials worthy of that name on human subjects.

Today, the drug tests are done according to the directions laid down by Stuebler, Mezger and H. Schulz (in Germany):

1 The nature of the drug under investigation is known only to the person in charge of the drug test. Double blind trials are not

acceptable, as the person in charge has a responsibility towards the subjects. He needs to have a rough idea of the potential risks. Other factors to be taken into account are the individual reactivity and receptiveness of subjects, increasing or attenuating the dose accordingly. When the drug under investigation is quite unknown, the person in charge will in any case be 'blind'.

2   The actual test period is preceded, interspersed or followed with placebo periods. Some subjects receive nothing but placebo. These safety factors increase the scientific validity of the test. They serve to differentiate between symptoms due to the drug and those due to the subject's expectations. Hahnemann had already arrived at many of the conclusions formed in pressent-day placebo research. He frequently resorted to intermittent doses of lactose.

3   The subjects should be in good health before and during the drug test. This is to prevent morbid changes obscuring or distorting the drug symptoms. A subject developing an intercurrent illness is excluded from the test, or an entry is made in the record so that these symptoms may be considered separately.

4   The age and sex distribution of subjects should be as wide as possible, to cover differences in response to the drug in question.

5   Subjects are asked to keep a diary in which all subjective and objective changes are noted down. Details concerning place, time, the specific nature of the change noted and dependence on environmental factors should be as accurate as possible.

6   The person in charge of the drug test will use clinical parameters such as ESR, blood and urine analysis, biochemical studies, ECG, temperature, pulse, blood pressure etc. to confirm objective signs.

7   The International Homoeopathic Medical League conducts worldwide multicentre drug tests. These eliminate climatic and racial differences from the test results and help to bring out the pure drug action which on the whole is uniform.

TOXICOLOGY AND PHARMACOLOGY

Drug tests on human subjects have their limits for 'humane' reasons. For obvious reasons it is not possible to ingest toxic materials in massive doses or over an extended period of time. The drug tests are therefore limited to the subtoxic range. Schoeler referred to this region as the 'fine toxicology'.[2] In this range, symptoms are largely subjective, consisting of changes experienced by the subject. Toxicology and pharmacology supply the data comprising objective signs and tissue changes.

Data from deliberate (forensic medicine) and accidental poisoning (accidents, industrial medicine) relate to the organic lesions and profound functional disorders a particular substance may cause.

Plato gave an accurate description of Socrates's death from hemlock (*Conium maculatum*) poisoning.[3] Ascending paralysis caused by a toxic dose of hemlock juice cannot be reproduced in drug tests on healthy human subjects. The total spectrum of drug-induced disease covers everything from changes felt only subjectively, organic and functional disorders to a lethal outcome. Toxicology is a rich source of information here.

Example

Poisoning due to mercury taken by mouth produces definite changes in the mouth, stomach, rectum and kidneys.

Mouth: Marked salivation, offensive, stinking odour, gums swollen and ulcerated, tongue enlarged and showing imprint of teeth. Tonsils grow inflamed and show ulcerative tissue breakdown with pseudomembranes. We use these signs of massive poisoning as indications for the treatment of stomatitis, pseudomembranous angina and possibly also diphtheria (mercury cyanide). The intestine, and particularly the rectum, show ulcerations and inflammation. Stools are mixed with mucus and blood and there is marked tenesmus. Dysentery and ulcerative colitis may present with very similar symptoms. The objective signs in the intestine may be so much the same that it is impossible to decide on post-mortem examination (as Virchow himself pointed out) 'whether in a particular instance this is a serious case of dysentery or an equally serious one of mercury poisoning.'[4]

In cases of chronic mercury poisoning (e.g. due to exposure at work) mental symptoms also develop. They range from initial hyperactivity with motor and mental unrest to the final states of lethargy and dementia.

Trembling and even definite tremor are common. Flaccid paralysis is also frequently seen. The skin reacts with many different types of efflorescence that resemble the skin lesions seen with secondary syphilis — a disease capable of imitating almost every dermatological condition. The resemblance between the symptoms of syphilis and those of mercury poisoning is altogether remarkable. Mercury was therefore the remedy of choice in the treatment of syphilis for many centuries.

In 1845, Zlatorovic, Professor at the Medical School in Vienna, was going through the actions of mercury in one of his lectures when he suddenly realized how closely the description he was giving resembled the symptomatology of syphilis. This sudden insight made such an impact that he stopped his lecture, went home and took up the study of homoeopathy, a subject he had only known vaguely from hearsay until then.[5]

Mercury unfortunately also yields rich pickings when we consider all the things so prettily presented as 'side effects' today. Someone should have told those medicinal compounds what they are 'permitted' to do and what a pharmacologist would consider 'improper' in a drug-induced disease.

I should like to define the side effects of drugs more precisely in three respects:

1 They are more frequent and powerful the higher the toxic dose.
2 They depend on the patient's sensitivity (idiosyncrasy, allergy, prior exposure).
3 Drug actions are by nature always broader in spectrum than the indication set by man (desired curative effect).

Hahnemann has so far been the only one to draw the logical conclusion from these well-established facts:

1 He reduced the dose to a minimum.
2 The minimum dose is individually adapted to the patient's increased sensitivity.
3 The drug action must correspond to the totality of symptoms and signs in the individual case.

That is the only way in which the criteria of the Law of Similars can be met. Partial similarity is merely an apparent similarity and therefore inadequate to meet the criteria for effective homoeopathic treatment.

Example
On the surface many cases of tonsillitis resemble the inflammation and suppuration, and possibly also formation of pseudomembranes, seen with oral mercury poisoning. The crude toxicology is very much the same, but it will be necessary to go into the fine toxicology based on drug tests on healthy human subjects if the true picture is to emerge on which the choice of drug may be based. It is the true picture because it makes it possible to differentiate a particular tonsillitis from others that may appear similar. Essential criteria for a sore throat calling for mercury are:

i) Local changes corresponding to the toxic effects of mercury.
ii) Constricting, lancinating pain. Throat sensitive to touch. Breath smells foul.
iii) Profuse oily perspiration, does not relieve.
iv) Everything worse at night, particularly restless anxiety.
v) Heat aggravates, irrespective of whether in form of hot compresses to the throat, hot drinks or a hot room. On the other hand the patient does not like it very cold and on the whole tends to be chilly. Extremes of temperature are disliked.

The above example demonstrates the realistic value of drug tests on healthy human subjects and the importance of observing the patient under treatment. Only a successful cure can confirm the validity of data from both sources, providing differentiation from the crude toxicological signs which show superficial similarity.

CLINICAL DATA (*ex usu in morbis*)

Clinical use thus provides verification through positive results and clearly establishes genuine similarities. Beyond this, it yields additional data on drug actions.

Example

A woman with acne conglobata was given *Bromium*. The indication of *Bromium* for certain types of acne is based on the toxicology and the clinical use of the drug. In the past, epileptics were given high doses of bromine over extended periods for their sedative effect. Acne would often develop as a 'side effect' in these cases.

The patient's acne was soon cured. But because the *Bromium* had been so effective she continued to take it — for safety's sake, as she said. Four weeks later she came back to the surgery complaining of lancinating pains in her index finger. The finger was quite normal in appearance, there had been no trauma, movement was not restricted — n.a.d. Yet the subjective complaint of a patient who had to be believed could not be argued away. T. F. Allen's *Encyclopaedia of Pure Materia Medica* (vol. 2, p. 244) lists exactly the same pain under *Bromium*: 'Severe burning stitches in the tip of the left index finger' (symptom no. 660). This, then, was the explanation. Taking *Bromium* for an extended period, the patient had done an involuntary drug test and produced the symptom of pain in her finger. When the *Bromium* was discontinued the pain disappeared within eight days (*sic*).

VETERINARY USE

'Animal experiments' are done every day by veterinary surgeons using homoeopathy in so far as they are treating animals. There is of course no specific intention to do research and explore specific questions. Yet in a field where treatment has to be cost effective (particularly in the case of cattle and valuable riding horses) these 'experiments' are fully on a par with any other form of experiment and show how ridiculous it is to call homoeopathic therapy 'suggestive.' Treatment given to animals provides important data on drug actions, for the most these patients can do to express their subjective opinions is the wagging of a tail. It is the objective result which counts in this field. The therapeutic element contributed by the practitioner is entirely marginal. Wolter[6] has carried out double blind trials to demonstrate the differentiated action of *Caulophyllum* 30x in farrowing sows and the drug pictures of *Flor de piedra* in cows. Experimental animal studies have also been done to demonstrate the efficacy of homoeopathic drugs.[7] Many homoeopathic physicians have serious doubts as to the justification of animal experiments, feeling that man should not abuse helpless creatures. According to press reports, 10-12 million animals are used annually for questionable experiments in the FRG. Those responsible have been keeping silent.

Summary
Homoeopathy obtains data relating to drug actions from four sources:
— Drug tests on healthy human subjects
— Toxicology and pharmacology
— Clinical use
— Veterinary use, data obtained in veterinary medicine.

2 The Drug Picture
The term 'drug picture' has been used in the last chapter. It will be new to you, for the combination of 'drug' and 'picture' is not used in allopathic pharmacology. You are, however, familiar with the term 'clinical picture' in the field of pathology. It serves to describe the totality of symptoms presenting in a particular case.

Having 'broached' the four sources of drugs data we know the value which attaches to each of them. The knowledge we have from these sources provides the material we need to draw the 'drug picture'. This is a synthesis of all the individual bits of information; it is all the actions of a drug taken together, and it is a unity, a whole. 'Picture', 'unity' or 'whole' are terms used in the field of phenomenology. When it is a question of describing wholes and getting a mental picture of them, the cause-effect type of thinking is no longer adequate. Unfortunately today's medical profession knows practically nothing but the causal relations postulated by scientists. It is becoming evident at the present time that major potential insights are lost, that we are losing out, if thousands of years of human effort to gain philosophical insight are 'forgotten'. Universities have become places of education lacking in *universitas*. The materialistic science of biology of the nineteenth and twentieth centuries has reduced medicine like everything else to a onesided physical science based on causal explanation and fixed experimental data. [8]

The soul was then gradually allowed back into orthodox medicine through the 'backdoor'. Everything which has to do with soul and spirit is not open to causal explanation, it is phenomenon. In the same way there can be no causal explanation for the similarity relating drug picture and clinical picture.

Cause and effect are replaced by the inference If — Then. *If* the drug picture and the clinical picture of the individual patient are comparable on the basis of similarity, *then* the supposition is that this drug will cure that particular patient.

A strict cause-effect relationship is almost never found in the sphere of biology. Exaggerating slightly one might say that the classical laws of physics, however exact, do call for many boundary conditions. The experiment has to run in a vacuum if it is to meet the conditions that will give validity to the law of falling bodies. Biological experiments cannot be carried out in empty space, however. Any effort to cure a patient is an 'experiment' run under highly complex conditions. These conditions tend to remain impenetrable, unless the Law of Similars is applied. If we take the point that homoeopathy is a form of regulatory therapy, it is evident that the healing stimulus must be similar in nature to the stimulus that triggered the disease if there is to be the potential for a change of direction at the centre of regulation. A relation based on similarity between the actions of a drug and the individual clinical picture therefore has scientific logic. Bayr's working hypothesis of a cybernetic control circuit provides a plausible explanation for the Law of Similars.

Application of the Law of Similars presupposes that comparison is made between two wholes. It is therefore imperative that we combine all individual data on drug action to form a single drug picture.

The drug then achieves individuality, its actions forming a whole. Paracelsus spoke of medicinal agents in similarly holistic terms.[9] In the language used by homoeopathic physicians identification of drug picture and the image presented by the patient goes so far that they may speak of a *Pulsatilla* woman, a *Calcarea carbonica* child, a *Hyoscyamus* cough or *Arsenicum* fear. Phenomenological comparison has shown that certain types of person go particularly well with specific drug pictures. The name of the drug picture may then serve to describe such a type. We talk of the *Nux vomica* type, the *Phosphorus* type etc. It should be noted that only a limited number of deep-acting drugs permit comparison with types of people. They are chiefly elements and salts incorporated in body structures.[10]

Hahnemann did not yet use the term 'drug picture'. He wrote:

> The sum and essence of the morbid elements a drug is able to produce will only come close to being complete if based on a great number of observations made on many different subjects of both sexes who are suitable. (*Organon of Practical Medicine* § 135)

'The sum and essence of the morbid elements a drug is able to produce' — this is a concept we need to hold on to firmly in homoeotherapy, remembering that the 'sum and essence' is more than the sum of individual items of information.

Summary

The drug picture encompasses the individual items of information on drug action. Comparing drug action and the symptoms presented by the patient as two complete pictures is a phenomenological process. Hahnemann did not however use the term 'drug picture'. His holistic concept of drug action is expressed by the term 'sum and essence'.

3 Sources and Manufacture of Homoeopathic Drugs

Hahnemann was not only a medical genius, he was also an outstanding chemist, pharmacologist and pharmacist. In line with the professional ethos of pharmacologists and pharmacists he was pedantically accurate. His directions for the preparation of homoeopathic medicines are valid to this day and stand up to all scientific scrutiny. He was a real 'Mr Milligramme' — as we used to call the pharmacists among us in my student days. He was more than just exact and meticulously accurate, however, for he developed from scratch a completely new system of pharmacy. His era was scarcely able to provide the techniques to meet his standards and he therefore prepared all his medicines himself. He would gather his own herbs wherever possible or make his own extracts. He wanted to be sure his raw materials were genuine and in perfect condition. He took his pharmacy so seriously that there was no room for anything casual or for 'guestimates'. His critics would do well to realize that no physician before or after Hahnemann was as thorough, dedicated and farsighted in his work on the study and manufacture of drugs.

The raw materials for homoeopathic drugs come from all the kingdoms of nature (plant, animal, mineral), some are synthetic chemical compounds. Hahnemann himself developed new chemical compounds or new methods of preparing known compounds (*Calcarea carbonica Hahnemanni, Mercurius solubilis Hahnemanni*). He was the first to discover the colloidal solubility of substances insoluble in the crude state. In more recent times, morbid matter has also come to be used as the raw material for 'nosodes'. These include *Tuberculinum Koch exotoxin, Diphtherinum* and blood taken from the patient. The above examples show that homoeopathy is wide-ranging, young and modern as it continues to develop, with no intention of resting on its laurels. Hahnemann is no 'sacred cow' where we are concerned. He continued to do further research and improve on his work till the end of his life, and his successors continue to be active. Valuable new discoveries are taken up and integrated.

Every new edition of the German Homoeopathic Pharmacopoeia contains new developments. In the case of the 1979 edition this meant the inclusion of new detection methods such as spectral analysis etc. Following the directions given by Hahnemann, raw materials are processed to essences, tinctures, solutions or triturations.

Essence: The raw material consists in the fresh juice expressed from whole plants or parts of plants (flowers, leaves). 90% alcohol is added as a preservative.

Tincture: The raw material consists in powdered dried plant materials or crushed materials of animal origin (bees, ants etc.). 90-60% alcohol is used to extract the drug constituents by maceration or percolation.

Solution: The raw materials are mostly soluble salts and acids. Depending on their solubility, they are dissolved in water or alcohol.

Trituration: The raw material consists in insoluble minerals or finely powdered dried plant material (whole plants, roots, seeds, etc.). Preparation consists in trituration with lactose in a mortar for at least 1 hour.

The liquid starting materials (essences, tinctures, solutions) are collectively called *mother tinctures*. These and the original triturations of solids are designated by the symbol Ø. A *Pulsatilla* mother tincture for instance is prescribed as *Pulsatilla* Ø. Gold in its original trituration is known to apothecaries as *Aurum trit.* Ø.

Homoeopathic medicines are dispensed as drops, tablets, pills, powders and granules. Ointments and glycerin-based mixtures are available for external and ampoules for parenteral use.

For prescribing purposes, the following abbreviations are used:

dil.	= **dilution**	= **solution**	
tabl.	= **tablet**		
trit.	= **trituration**	= **powder**	
glob.	= **globuli**	= **granules**[11]	

The choice depends on the starting material and the needs of the individual patient. Materials which are insoluble in their original form (e.g. gold) can only be prepared as tablets or trituration in the low potency range (generally anything below 8x). Others which are liquid, like bromine, and present a hazard to the pharmacist if triturated with lactose due to contact with air and the heat of friction) have to be prescribed as a dilution up to 8x. Beyond that point they may be prescribed in any form.

Tablets are preferable to solutions when travelling. Children will sometimes refuse to take alcoholic solutions. This is why granules are dispensed. Children will readily take these for they are made of cane sugar. They are medicated with the prescribed solution and then dried. The potency label given to granules refers to the solution which has been applied to them. The influence of the small quantity of cane sugar is negligible in this respect.

Summary
Homoeopathic medicines derive from the plant, animal and mineral kingdoms. A few are based on synthetic compounds. Those prepared from morbid matter are known as nosodes.

Homoeopathic pharmacy was developed by Hahnemann himself. His work has been so accurate that, except for technical refinements, the German Homoeopathic Pharmacopoeia still follows his directions.

Processing with water or alcohol produces solutions, essences or tinctures. These are collectively referred to as mother tinctures and designated Ø.

The abbreviations used in prescribing different presentations are:

liquid		= dil.
dry	— powder	= trit.
	— tablet	= tab.
	— granule	= glob.

4 Potentization
During the early stages, when he was still feeling his way, Hahnemann gave the drugs in measurable quantities, without processing them further. He noted, however, that giving drugs in the traditional form was not the best way. Depending on the nature of the original material the drug reaction tended to be too powerful (side effects, excessive initial reaction, marked initial aggravation) or it was inadequate because the material had not been suitably prepared (particularly in the case of insoluble minerals).

The logical conclusion was to develop a method for the processing of drugs that would give the best results in terms of quality as well as quantity. Hahnemann had also noted that there was individual variation in sensitivity and reactivity to drugs. The form of medical practice he advocated was designed to take account of the way reactions to a drug varied from individual to individual.

This was a clearly defined, rational goal. He achieved it by reducing the dose to a minimum and enhancing drug action by processing (trituration and succussion). This gave optimum medicinal power and avoided harmful effects. Hahnemann called these preparations potencies or dynamizations (*potentia* = power in the sense of ability, capacity; *dynamis* = power in the sense of strength). He called the process used to prepare his medicines potentization, a term, by the way, which he did not use before 1827.[12] The late date serves to indicate that he developed the method only after a long period of careful observation. It had to meet his high standards for the medicinal powers of drugs. In 1839 he wrote:

> Homoeopathic dynamizations genuinely bring to life the medicinal properties which lie hidden in natural solids when these are in the crude state.[13]

As modern physicians we do not normally make up and dispense our own medicines, and our colleagues in conventional medicine know little of the mysteries in the chemist's retort. When it comes to homoeopathic medicines, however, it is essential that we have accurate knowledge of their origin and manufacture. There are threats on the horizon. Even today, certain potencies are no longer obtainable in the FRG because of drugs regulations (e.g. *Cannabis indica, Coca*).

PREPARATION AND DEGREE OF DILUTION
Liquid formulations based on the mother tincture are mixed by 10 firm downward succussions for each stage of potentization.

At each stage, dilution with the vehicle (water, alcohol, lactose) is in a ratio of 1:9 (decimal scale, designated by a small letter 'x') or 1:99 (centesimal scale, designated by a small 'c').

Hahnemann used the centesimal scale until late in life (Paris). In his last years he developed a method of potentizing with sugar granules. The resulting potencies are known as 50,000th or LM potencies.[14] Constantin Hering (1800-80, German-born physician, emigrated to USA) used the decimal scale to potentize snake venoms, and Vehsemeier gave a more detailed description of this scale in 1836.

Today, all three scales are used, though the LM potencies relatively seldom. In France the centesimal scale is exclusively used, in English-speaking countries predominantly the centesimal scale, and in Germany on the whole the decimal scale (designated D1 etc. in German-speaking countries).

Both the centesimal and the decimal scale have their protagonists. In my own experience (unsupported by statistical analysis) the decimal scale is better for low potencies up to 6x, whilst the centesimal scale provides more rapidly acting medicines in the higher potencies. The anthroposophical school of medicine stresses — no doubt rightly — that the number of potentizing stages is more important than the ratio between medicinal agent and vehicle.[15] In the case of decimal potencies, the number of potentizing stages is twice that of comparable centesimal potencies. Such a comparison based on pure arithmetic undoubtedly has validity only with regard to the amount of original medicinal substance present in the low potencies. Thus a 3c potency corresponds to the 6x, a 6c to the 12x.

The German Homoeopathic Pharmacopoeia gives detailed directions in every case. Here is an example taken from p. 21, concerning the potentization of fluids:

> The potentization of fluids requires a room protected from direct sun light. The vials used must have a capacity ½ to ⅓ times greater than the volume to be potentized. The name of the drug and the number of the potency for which the vial is to be used should be written on the cork as well as the vial itself, using a capital C followed by the number for centesimal potencies and a capital D for decimal potencies. [German notation; C1 = 1c in English, D1 = 1x. Translator.] Potentization is effected by using proportional volumes for large quantities and drops for small quantities.
>
> Having been labelled with the name of the drug and numbered C1 — C30, as described above, the vials are placed on the table in sequence and 99 parts of ethyl alcohol put in each from the C2 upwards, using a measuring cylinder. The first centesimal potency is made up from the essence, tincture or solution, as defined in the individual paragraphs and transferred to the C1 vial.

The paragraphs referred to above give exact instructions for the preparation of 1c (or 1x) potencies. This differs slightly depending on the nature of the raw material. The amount of sap varies from plant to plant, the solubility of salts differs, and extracts made from matter of animal origin also vary. The end result is that every 1c or 1x potency contains medicinal sustance and alcohol in a ratio of 1:99 and 1:9 respectively, the total amount always being 100 and 10 parts respectively.

> One part from the 1c vial is then transferred to the 2c vial, the latter is stoppered and its contents mixed by applying ten firm downward succussions. Then one part of the contents of vial 2c is transferred to vial 3c, the latter is succused ten times to give the 3c potency, and potentization continues like this, always transferring one part of the preceding potency to the next vial in sequence and succussing ten times.

This illustrates the basic principle of potentization. A corresponding method is used to potentize dry materials with lactose as the vehicle.

MULTIPLE OR SINGLE VIAL POTENCIES

Every potency has to be produced in a new vial, yet many of the intermediate potencies are never used. The proper method is therefore expensive. Hahnemann always used it, though he tended not to be well off financially. It is known as Hahnemann's Multiple Vial Method. The French are very accurate in calling potencies produced by this method CH 1, 2, 3 etc.

Single vial potencies are easier and cheaper to produce. The disadvantage is that they are less accurate. They are called Korsakoff potencies, the method having been developed by the Russian General Korsakoff.

His method is based on the fact that when a vial is emptied some of the fluid remains adhering to the walls. You have emptied a glass of red wine — but is it really empty? When it has stood for a while a small amount of wine will have collected at the bottom of the glass. Korsakoff did careful weighing tests and found that one drop will on average remain when a vial has been emptied 'by shaking out the contents with a firm downward stroke of the arm'. There will be variation in the amount left behind depending on the nature of the glass walls (may vary with different manufactures) and the surface tension of the starting material. Hahnemann's method was and still is more accurate. Whatever one's reservations, the efficacy of Korsakoff potencies is good, however. If we take the view that the number of potentizing steps is more important than the ratio of medicinal agent to vehicle the Korsakoff method has much to be said for it, requiring less effort and expenditure. Potentization is continuous, using one and the same vial, the residue remaining when the vial is emptied providing the starting material for the next potency. The method is very useful for the manufacture of centesimal potencies above the 30c. The German Homoeopathic Pharmacopoeia does not include it.

Summary

Hahnemann found that medicinal substances were often not sufficiently active in the crude, unprocessed state and that the doses used by his predecessors and contemporaries were too large. Drug processing (trituration, succussion) and reduction of the dose gave optimum results as regards both quality and quantity. He called his method potentization. The medicines produced by it were called potencies or dynamizations. Potencies are produced on the decimal (1 + 9 = 10) and centesimal (1 + 99 = 100) scale. During his last years, Hahnemann also evolved a method of potentization with sugar granules; the resulting potencies are called LM potencies.

The method of potentization given in the German Homoeopathic Pharmacopoeia requires a new vial to be used for every stage of potentization, which is the original method developed by Hahnemann. Another method, using only a single vial, was introduced by Korsakoff.

1. Vonessen, F. used this as the title for his profound medicophilosophical treatise on mythical equivalence concepts, Aristotle's catharsis and the concept of practical homoeopathic medicine.

2. Schoeler, H. *Ueber angewandte Toxikologie.*

3. Plato's deeply moving report is probably the oldest 'drug test' with a toxic dose on record. For a translation (German), see Charette, p. 194.

4. Schulz, H. [1956] p. 308.

5. Charette, p. 316.

6. Wolter, in Gebhardt, K. H. *Beweisbare Homöopathie.*

7. Plentiful material in Wurmser, L. *Die Entwicklung der homöopathischen Forschung.*

8. Bamm, *Ex Ovo.* p. 142ff.

9. For comparison between Paracelsus and homoeopathy, see Clarke, J. H. 1923; Schultz, C. H. 1831.

10. Beuchelt [1956].

11. Where forms are concerned terminology can be confusing. It should be noted that English 'pills' are known as 'granules' overseas, whilst English 'granules' are referred to as 'globuli' overseas. See Ainsworth, J. B. L. Homoeopathic pharmacy. The present state of the art. *Br Hom J* 1983; **72**:163. — Translator.

12. Comment to be found in Tischner, *Das Werden der Homöopathie.*

13. *Chronic Diseases* vol. 5, Preface. See also *Organon* § 270.

14. *Organon*, p. 270. To the best of my knowledge, Flury first drew attention to this new method of dynamization in *Realitätserkenntnis und Homöopathie*, p. 63 [Engl. *Homoeopathy and the Principle of Reality*, pp. 52-3].

15. Anthroposophical medicine has done a considerable amount of work on problems relating to potentization. For a good review, see Itschner, V., and others.

4
SYMPTOMATOLOGY

A patient's symptoms point the way to the drug he needs. Homoeopathy specifically treats the individual and therefore takes into account not only disease-specific (pathognomic) but also the more important subject-specific symptoms.

Symptoms provide information on the aetiology and localization of a disorder and also on the changes the patient experiences in body, soul and spirit. It is important to establish factors that influence the patient and the times when they do so (modalities).

In Chapter III we considered the basic principles of pharmacology. We have identified the sources of our knowledge relating to drug actions. We are aware of the significance of the drug picture and we know how homoeopathic medicines are manufactured and potentized.

This chapter will consider the symptomatology of the patient. Symptoms are phenomena in ourselves and others which we see, hear, feel, smell and detect by using special methods of investigation. In short, we perceive them with all our sense organs. The phenomena we observe need not necessarily be pathological. It is only when several phenomena occur in conjunction or a single phenomenon grows over-powering that we must rate this an alarm signal to indicate pathology.

On principle, no particular value should attach to any phenomenon and it should be considered entirely neutral. None should be excluded and none given undue weight. Modern school medicine is onesided in this respect. The only symptoms which count are those that fit into the anatomical and/or physiological pathology of a particular disease concept. Hahnemann insisted that the totality of symptoms was always to be condidered. The totality (synthesis) of symptoms is obtained by history-taking, observation and examination. A certain order will emerge on evaluation of the total material (analysis). This order is based on the hierarchic order of the person: phenomena relating to soul and spirit come before those relating to the body; anything relating to the whole person comes before local symptoms; anything specific to the individual is rated higher than anything one would normally expect to see with a particular disease.

One more thing we must be clear about: our primary aim is not to remove symptoms. Homoeopathy never is and never has been a 'symptom cover-up'. Homoeopathy is concerned with treating ill-health from the roots, and not with the removal of individual symptoms. It is a causal form of therapy.

The aim of homoeopathic treatment is not to remove or suppress a symptom by any direct route. That is the aim of official pharmacology when used palliatively (analgesics for pain, laxatives for constipation). Gathering all the symptoms (totality of symptoms) of the sick person by taking the history, observing and examining the patient serves only one purpose — to find the right and most similar medicine. This will stimulate autoregulation and achieve 'the rapid, gentle, and lasting restoration of health.' (*Organon* § 2).

Example
An infant with milk crusts would not be treated with local applications to the skin. The totality of symptoms may show intolerance of cow's milk with intestinal problems, head sweats, retarded development, signs of rickets. This total picture corresponds to *Calcarea carbonica*. This medicine can cure the accompanying symptoms and the milk crusts.

Symptoms reflect the inner nature of the disease to the outside, so that a homoeopathic physician is able to interpret it:

Symptoms point the way in the search for the drug which will initiate recovery in the individual case.

Symptoms also provide information on the stage a disease has reached. Objective clinical symptoms are preceded by the patient feeling unwell. This enables homoeopathic physicians to give treatment on the basis of such early symptoms, whilst allopathic medicine has to wait until a diagnosis can be made and laboratory reports are available.

1 Totality of Symptoms
You will recall that the Law of Similars — *similia similibus* — requires the physician to determine the drug which is capable of evoking changes similar to the symptoms the patient presents with. The drug showing greatest similarity is chosen by comparing the range of symptoms evoked by the drug with the patient's symptomatology.

Changes experienced by healthy subjects exposed to the drug are given verbal expression; functional changes (eliminations, peripheral vascular changes etc.) may also occur. Toxicology provides further data concerning changes and lesions in tissues and organs capable of objective assessment. All these data together make up the drug picture. This is matched against the totality of symptoms presenting in the patient.

It has to be stressed that two *wholes* are compared. Primitive symptom cover-ups are not homoeopathy.

Totality of symptoms — what does it mean? The 'sum of symptoms' is a sum of individual items collected without attaching particular value to any. The term 'totality of symptoms' on the other hand expresses the holistic approach to disease practised in homoeopathy, with individual data assigned a value within the whole. 'The whole does not consist in parts *being* together, but in their *acting* together.' (Leeser)

2 Symptoms of Disease and Patient
Pathognomic and Personal Symptoms

The symptoms a patient reports and those we uncover on observation and examination are a motley mixture. We bring order into the melée by dividing them into two groups. The first group serves to establish the clinical diagnosis, the disease (pathognomic symptoms). The second group (personal symptoms) reflect the patient's individual reactivity to pathogenic factors.

Examples

1   Mother's report on a house visit:

'My daughter has been running a temperature for 4 days now. At first her eyes were a bit sensitive to light and reddened and she had a running nose. She then developed a hollow-sounding cough. This morning I noted a red rash behind her ears and in the course of the day this has spread over the face and chest.

'She has been rather tearful since she's been ill. I keep asking her if she has a pain anywhere. No, nothing hurts. And immediately she's crying again. She is normally a cheerful child. Now she lies there patiently. Today she asked for the heating to be turned off, she'd rather have the room cool — I had thought I must make sure she does not catch a chill, seeing she is not well.'

The first group of symptoms were pathognomic and directly led to the diagnosis of measles.

The child's tearfulness and patient attitude and the desire for a cool room do not directly relate to the disease. These were definitely personal reactions, on the basis of which *Pulsatilla* was the drug of choice for the homoeopathic physician.

2   A woman was complaining of bouts of headaches over a period of 20 years. Attacks were preceded by flickering in front of the eyes, she would be

feeling miserably sick and have to vomit. She needed quiet and darkness — that would be best. When the pain was at its height she had to urinate copiously, producing very pale urine. After this, she felt better.

The diagnosis based on these symptoms was migraine. Detailed questioning revealed that she used to be highly irascible in the past but had learned to control herself. The headache went from the forehead to behind the nose and deep inside, causing nausea and also vomiting. Repertorization based on these personal symptoms — irascible and pain moving towards the nose — showed *Agaricus* to be the homoeopathic drug of choice. This cured a migraine of 20 years standing.

Comment: in the second case, the obvious, pathognomic symptoms related only to the diagnosis. It needed the personal symptoms to arrive at a drug which the characteristic migraine pattern had not led one to consider. *Gelsemium* matched the pathognomic symptoms. I had given this drug first (very wrong, I confess), without result. Failure did however lead to careful history-taking, paying due attention to personal symptoms, and ultimate success.

These two examples demonstrate clearly why Hahnemann was always asking for cases to be considered on an individual basis. Faithful adherence to this does pay dividends. 'Do as I do, but properly so' — unfortunately the apprentices often think they know better than the master. Section 153 of the *Organon* tells us how to do it.

SIGNIFICANCE OF PERSONAL SYMPTOMS
(*Organon* § 153)

Slightly abbreviated, § 153 of Hahnemann's *Organon of Practical Medicine* (6th edition) says: 'In choosing the homoeopathic drug specific to the case, particular and almost exclusive attention must be given to the more remarkable, peculiar, unusual and singular (characteristic) signs and symptoms . . .'

This is the point on which everything turns whenever we are looking for the appropriate drug. Section 153 is perfectly clear, simple and logical. Unfortunately it tends to be misunderstood, reinterpreted by those who think they know better, or forgotten. Fanatics also tend to attach legendary importance to it. Yet its real value lies in commonsense realization and the practical need to find *distinguishing* characteristics that will isolate a particular set of circumstances from a host of circumstances. Analogous to this, the criminologist will look for a finger print to provide proof of the criminal's identity.

The disease label is a collective term, distinguishing marks are only to be found by considering individual reactions.

I do not recognize a particular person because he or she has two arms and two legs; it is their peculiar gait, their uniquely individual gestures, some particular characteristic which will identify one individual among a thousand others.

In political cartoons, a few strokes of the pen characterize an individual so well that millions will recognize him. Such recognition is possible only on the basis of remarkable, peculiar and unusual individual characteristics.

Section 153 is so important that it forces us to consider the terms 'remarkable, peculiar, unusual and singular' individually.

Life does not go according to paragraphs and design, and the above terms often overlap. Something which is remarkable will often also be unusual, and much that is unusual will also be remarkable. There is no point in applying the philologist's dissecting knife to these terms. Let us go to the patient and get a concrete idea of what Hahnemann was after.

A patient had *remarkably* red ears. It was not frostbite, nor was there any local lesion. His lips were also very red. He had a bit of a running nose and the nasal orifices were red. All body orifices were remarkably red.

The *peculiar* thing with this patient was that he had diarrhoea driving him from his bed at about 6 a.m.; not during the day, not at night, — this sudden urge to stool and diarrhoea occurred only in the mornings.

The following statement made by the patient also ranks as peculiar: 'I get annoyed at anything. A single word can make me wild and I lose control.' This really was worth noting in so far as the overall impression he gave was one of self-control and his profession (in banking) had trained him to be pleasant to people.

Something *unusual* for an active personality full of the joys of life was the following, told to me by his wife who said that he was very despondent at times; he might sit there brooding, wringing his hands, with the whole future looking bleak to him.

The patient consulted me for rheumatoid arthritis. The wrists showed marked swelling. Asked as to whether there was any pain, he said impulsively: 'Pain — there are no words to describe it. It burns like fire. I get the same burning pain around the anus. First there is terrible irritation and when I start scratching the itching stops and there is this burning pain. The anus gets really bad on contact with water. I can't take a bath at all, only a shower. I take care to avoid water getting near it. I use oil to keep my backside clean.' Burning pain, irritation changing to burning when scratched, worse from water — those are singular, characteristic symptoms of *Sulphur*.

CONCOMITANT SYMPTOMS

Patients will often report pain or functional disorders occurring elsewhere in the body *at the same time* as their main complaint. The principal complaint is accompanied by another sensation.

Example

For years, Mr KM complained of occasional bouts of pain in the region of the two lowest left ribs. The history included renal calculi being passed, the last time 3 years previously, and elevated uric acid levels. His previous doctor had therefore put him on long-term uricostatic therapy. Homoeopathic history-taking did not yield much, and there was no indication for a particular drug. He was therefore first of all given *Berberis* as an organotropic drug, unfortunately with no result. It was only when he came to see me for the fourth time that he mentioned — quite in passing — that he felt lightning-type stabbing pains in the right ear at times when there was pain also in the left flank. He was given *Natrum sulphuricum* and this got rid of the pain in the left flank and in the ear and also kept his uric acid levels normal.

Concomitant symptoms showing obvious connexion with the principal complaint are without significance in finding the appropriate drug — a headache accompanying a cold in the head for example. It is *remarkable* however if a woman reports diarrhoea accompanying her monthly periods; or toothache during the period yet her dentist can find no reason for this.

KEY SYMPTOMS

Key symptoms are nuggets of gold, and like all good things they are rare and not immediately obvious. If one knows the leading symptoms of drugs really well (these are particularly characteristic symptoms in the drug picture) it is possible to spot the real characteristics in among all the general signs and symptoms. The patient's key symptom corresponds to the leading symptom of the drug. It decodes the case. The key symptom, or rather symptoms, must be expressed with feeling by the patient, they must be clearly characteristic and should be complete symptoms (see Chapter 4, 4).

A single key symptom is not normally enough to base a prescription on, just as a single leading symptom does not define a drug. Lock and key provide an analogy: a crude key showing little differentiation will open quite a number of locks, a safe on the other hand can only be opened with one specific key. The more complex and complete the profile of a key symptom is, finding its match in a symptom expressed in his or her own words by someone taking part in a drug test, the surer can we be of it being the right one. It requires experience to judge the quality of the key and find the right lock.

Von Boenninghausen gave particular preference to key and concomitant symptoms in deciding on the appropriate drug. He used them to establish relationships between drugs. At the present time von Keller in Tuebingen, FRG, is doing skilful work with key symptoms and getting impressive results. He uses complete symptoms wherever possible.

Example
1   Telephone call from a worried mother at about midnight. 'My child has got ill very suddenly. He woke screaming from his sleep and has a high temperature. He's been out toboganning during the day. I expect he caught a cold in the cold, biting wind. What is really worrying me is that he is so afraid. It is almost impossible to calm him down. You know he is not normally subject to fears.'

Examination when I visited at home revealed no appreciable disease. What shocked me, however, was the sudden question: 'Do I have to go to hospital now? Will I have to die?'

This case clearly brought out a key symptom of *Aconitum*: Following exposure to cold winds, infection with sudden onset around midnight, skin hot and dry, remarkable fear, fear of having to die.

2   Student, female, aged 28, seen on 29 Sept. 1976.
'I have a headache again, it has been getting worse in the back of the neck, at the point where the neck joins the back of the head, and then somehow it is everywhere in my head; there is a feeling as though I ought to use counterpressure, tie a scarf around firmly because the head feels as if it is expanding, yet at the same time also as if it were too massive, as if it were condensing and as if I had to compress it. My stomach has also been playing up recently, sweets do not agree with me at all.' (From a tape recording, von Keller, Tuebingen)

Here we have a key symptom of *Argentum nitricum*: Headache from nape to back of head with sensation as if the head were too big. Better from pressure and firm bandaging. Concomitant symptoms: Desire for sweets which do not agree.

3 Objective and Subjective Symptoms —
Symptoms and Signs

In English medical language, objective evidence of disease is commonly referred to as 'signs'. This includes all data and parameters resulting from special investigations. The word 'symptom' is both an umbrella term and the term used for subjective sensations reported by the patient. Anything a physician sees, palpates or finds out from investigations is referred to as 'signs' or objective symptoms. Anything he hears from the patient or perceives intuitively comes under the heading of subjective symptoms. The distinction is of no particular significance. What matters is whether anything I see in a patient is what I would expect (e.g. a red rash in a case of measles) or unique to the individual (e.g. the red ears in the *Sulphur* case).

4 Complete Symptoms

'A stool needs at least three legs to stand securely.' A really useful symptom should also have at least three legs. A stool will stand even more firmly on four legs.

A complete symptom has four elements. It must have details as to aetiology and location. The nature of the sensation has to be described, and special conditions (modalities) have to be clearly established.

A patient points to the spot as he says: 'There is a sharp pain here in the right chest when I take a deep breath. The pain started after exposure to cold.' That is a complete symptom with clear statements as to aetiology, location, the nature of the sensation and special condition. The patient has in fact been describing the characteristic pain that calls for *Bryonia*.

When taking the history in homoeopathic medicine we must always do our best to obtain complete symptoms. With this goal in mind, it is often possible to put the questions that will help us to achieve it.

AETIOLOGY

It is not always possible to elicit the triggering factor in a case of illness, or the patient may be too imaginative in presenting it. But if the patient is really definite in saying: 'Since I fell off that ladder and got concussion I've been having these continuous headaches' — *Arnica* will probably help, particulary if other *Arnica* symptoms are present. Or else a painter and decorator may say that he got really frozen the day before yesterday when working in that newly built house and then the next day got cramp-like pain in the region of the sciatic nerve, had to lie in bed with his legs drawn up. *Colocynthis* will be the drug of choice in that case. A mother may report that her child got a serious fright, was more or less paralyzed for a time after that and has since been stammering. Here the aetiology points to a group of drugs that have 'complaint due to fright' (*Aconitum, Ignatia, Natrium muriaticum, Opium* and others). If a student suffers from an occipital headache after reading a lot, the aetiology suggests the need for an eye test before any drug is prescribed. The last example shows that asking for the triggering factor may also provide an answer as to the nature of the disorder, making it clear from the beginning what form of treatment — surgical, medical, dietary etc. — is indicated.

If definite aetiological symptoms are present, care must be taken not to lose track of them when looking for the appropriate drug. The aetiology often proves a safe route to the simile.

Kent's *Repertory* has the aetiological symptoms scattered through all its rubrics. In Dorcsi's *Symptomenverzeichnis* (index of symptoms) they are listed under 'Mental and physical trauma'. The term 'trauma' has to be taken in a somewhat wider sense. Any suppression of normal or pathological eliminations may also be considered under that heading. All the consequences of such suppression are considered among the group of 'aetiological factors'. External applications to skin lesions, a spray used to stop coryza, painting the feet to stop foot sweats, possibly also diarrhoea stopped with tincture of opium, infections curbed with powerful drugs, and many a hypermenorrhoea treated by D & C or surgically — all of these may give rise to sequelae. Modern treatments are often heroic and really need critical assessment with regard to their sequelae. Seeming success cannot satisfy physicians who are capable of thinking and observation and following up particular patients for extended periods of time. Passing the patient on from one specialist to another tends to prevent this type of observation in the present age. *Aude sapere*. Dare to think for yourself.

The subtly balanced steady state of the organism does not tolerate disruptive interventions. The most delicate clockwork is a crude piece of machinery compared to the balanced harmony of the organism. We do not like to a see a watchmaker working with a hammer and an axe.

The difficult issue of suppressive treatments reveals the real benefit to be obtained with homoeopathy: It is a gentle force. 'The highest ideal in medicine is the rapid, gentle and lasting restoration of health.' (*Organon* § 2)

LOCALIZATION

The localization of a complaint usually takes us into the sphere of clinical diagnosis. Local symptoms are often pathognomic. The drug tests have shown that many drugs have a preference for specific organs or tissues or interfere with specific functions. Many drugs show a definite organotropism or functiotropism. The relation of *Mercury* to the oral and anal mucosa has already been described; *Phosphorus* is known to affect the liver and kidneys; *Bryonia* attacks the serous membranes. These are just a few examples of specific relations to certain organs and tissues. Details as to localization can therefore lead to the pathognomic syndrome and finally the specific drug. Care must be taken, however, not to fall into the error of applying short-circuit therapy based on such local symptoms. There are certain well established indications which permit the right drug to be found with almost complete certainty on the basis of localization, but they are exceptions to the rule.[1] In daily practice, under pressure of time, these well-established indications can save an enormous amount of time. We are right to use them, but must in all honesty admit that this is a form of 'instant' homoeopathy. The stool wobbles; it has only one leg.

Examples
Gingivitis gravidarum always responds to *Mercurius solubilis*. Pain in the right thorax relating to respiration responds well to *Bryonia alba*. Cramp in the calf muscles disappears with *Cuprum aceticum*. Pain in abdominal muscle, particularly during pregnancy: *Bellis perennis*. Pain in the coccyx and adjacent areas (coccygodynia): *Castor equorum*.

In homoeopathy, our efforts must always be directed at producing a 'tailor-made suit'; off-the-peg goods are already flooding the market.

The third supporting pillar of homoeopathy is strict individualization in every single case. Prescribing on the clinical diagnosis only is a crime. So is prescribing on localization only. If anything it is palliative treatment; a genuine cure is achieved only by restoring autoregulation. This calls for the totality of symptoms, and the localization is part of that whole. The local symptom can often be differentiated further and made more drug-specific if a definite pattern emerges between lateralities of different symptoms or if there is a direction of movement. Most drugs organotropic to the liver and gallbladder for instance have right-sided local symptoms: *Chelidonium* has pain in the right supraorbital region and at the lower angle of the right scapula; with *Lycopodium* the right foot is warmer than the left; *Lachesis* has marked affinity with the left side of the body. Patients will often say: 'Funny — everything I've got is on the left — headache, tonsillitis, pains in the arm, mastitis, pain in the ovary —' (*Lachesis*). Or: 'Everything starts on the left and then moves to the right' (*Lachesis* and others). Others again will say: 'First everything is on the right, then all my problems migrate to the left' (*Lycopodium* and *Sulphur* among others).

Or a cross-over pattern may emerge: first the left shoulder hurts and then the right hip (*Ledum*). In Kent's *Repertory* the direction a pain is radiating is given under the heading 'extending to'. If patients come up with clear statements of this nature it is possible to select drugs from larger groups, providing the pain is not radiating from a gross organic lesion.

Summary

Local symptoms point to the organotropism and functiotropism of drugs.
They are often pathognomic and may relate to the clinical diagnosis.
This limits their value in determining the appropriate drug in a case.
A single local symptom will rarely be an adequate basis for individualized
therapy, though there are some notable exceptions. A local symptom
may be more clearly defined by details as to laterality and the direction
in which pain radiates.

SENSATION

We need to get the patient to describe the nature of the abnormal
sensation as accurately as possible. The power of the sensation is
particularly important in deciding on the weight which attaches to
the symptom. General statements such as 'It hurts' are not much help.
If there is pain, the patient should try and define the nature of the
pain. Simple, less sophisticated people often give very apt and descriptive
details: it burns like fire; sharp like a pin; it is thumping, I can feel a
pulse beating; my leg feels as if it was being tied up; the pain comes
shooting in like lightning. All symptoms described with 'as if' or 'as
though' tend to be highly individual. The group is referred to as the
'as if symptoms' in the literature. Sensations in the 'as if' group rank
highly. Such a way of putting it means that the patient is really
identifying with the sensation. Modern intellectuals unfortunately often
have scientific pretensions and do not use such descriptive terms.[2]

This is the age of half-informed magazine readers who tend to come
along with their ready-made diagnosis: 'Problems with the circulation'
— 'I've got a slipped disk'. It needs patience and tact, avoiding any hint
of superiority, to restore the patient to a state of 'innocence'. He will
be asked to tell, very simply, how it feels to him and what he has
observed. To find the appropriate drug we need personal symptoms
and not half-understood half-knowledge. Above all we are looking for
sensations involving the whole body. It has been said, in the section
on localization, that details as to location may often lead to the diagnosis,
i.e. are pathognomic and of less value for individualization. Sensations
confined to part of the body are similarly limited in value. They are
of value if they meet the conditions given in the *Organon* § 153 —
being remarkable, peculiar, unusual and singular. Sensations felt
simultaneously in different parts of the body or involving the whole
person immediately carry greater weight. The whole ranks higher than
its parts. The human being is an indivisible whole. For purely practical
reasons, sensations are considered at three levels: mind, intellect and
body.

MIND, INTELLECT AND BODY

Symptoms relating to the patient's emotional state ('mind' symptoms or 'mentals') carry the greatest weight — providing they are clearly and precisely defined. Mental symptoms usually occur well ahead of all else when a pathological process is developing. Subjective sensations will almost always precede clinical evidence. Changes in the sphere of soul and spirit provide very early indications for homoeopathic treatment, long before functional or morphological changes are in evidence.

Mothers often tell us that their children are 'out of sorts' for two or three days before they develop an illness, being insufferable, aggressive or tearful. Early prevention is possible at this stage by giving the drug matching the changes at the emotional level. A tearful child will respond well to *Pulsatilla*; a vehement, furious child may be better for *Nux vomica* or *Bryonia*; one who is rather quiet and withdrawn for *Ignatia*; unsufferable, over-excited children need *Chamomilla*; sudden intense night-time fear responds to *Aconitum*.

There are definite stages of complexity in the organization of organisms. The higher life forms also have greater potential for bringing soul and spirit to expression. I am choosing my words carefully because recent discoveries (e.g. with Kirlian photography)[3] have demonstrated something which has really been known for a long time — that plants, too, have sensibilities (Fechner). The elements that distinguish man and differentiate between individual persons are most clearly apparent in the sphere of soul and spirit. Homoeopathy has its domain in everything that is individual and personal. This explains why so much weight attaches to emotional states in the practice of homoeopathy.

The homoeopathic materia medicas list changes in mental state for every drug. Once again Hahnemann was well ahead of his own and even the present time, for the concept of 'psychotropic drugs' has only come up recently.

The vast complex of **fear and anxiety,** a major element in human life, also comes to expression in the relevant drug pictures. This corroborates the holistic image of the human being as someone who plays his or her part, which is taken as a matter of course in homoeopathy. Concomitant symptoms in the physical sphere define and differentiate different fears and anxieties. Concomitant symptoms relating to the cardiovascular system for instance can visibly differentiate the 'red fear' of *Belladonna* and *Aurum* from the 'pale fear' of *Veratrum album* and *Arsenicum album*. Apprehensive fears (of examinations, a journey etc.) cause diarrhoea (*Argentum nitricum*); fear of thunderstorms will make otherwise perfectly sensible people hide under the stairs (*Phosphorus*); fear of animals and particularly dogs

(*Tuberculinum*); fear of being left on one's own (*Calcarea carbonica*); fear of being alone (*Arsenicum album*).

All symptoms connected with the most powerful of our instincts, that of the **preservation of life** — and the fear of death and dying which is another aspect of this — merit very careful attention. Destructive impulses to destroy or injure oneself, murderous impulses, hatred, extreme rage, unfounded jealousy, reckless extravagance, meanness, arrogance, feelings of superiority or inferiority — the whole rich variety of emotional reactions reflects the nature of the individual. As soon as they go beyond a certain limit of tolerance they rank as pathological and play a key role in choosing the appropriate drug.

Dreams reflect unconscious fears and longings. They will often yield valuable symptoms. Many functional disorders which at the surface appear to be purely physical are essentially reflecting mental suffering. Hahnemann's followers are very fortunate in so far as homoeopathic treatment brings to practical realization many of the things psychosomatic medicine has brought to light in recent years. Psychodynamics — a very modern-sounding concept — may be found in §§ 210-30 of Hahnemann's *Organon*, written 150 years ago.

For a physician who brings a certain acuity to his observation it can be almost as exciting as unravelling a murder mystery to 'read between the lines.' There is much the patient does not tell us. Fear will be masked by exaggeratedly lively high spirits or a gushing attitude; by an asthma attack or enuresis nocturna. Anger shows itself in biliary colics; hurt feelings in gastric ulcers. Fear meets us with cold, sweaty hands; persistent constipation may be due to reduced flow of bile, shock or extreme tight-fistedness. Old guilt feelings tend to be hidden; silence during a conversation can say much, a dismissive gesture explain a great deal. The more the patient feels that there is a helping hand reaching out to him, the nearer will his statements come to the truth. In the course of the interview the patient will often come to realize his own insincerity. He gradually feels able to let go of his camouflage. The search for the simile is not helped by camouflaged 'false' symptoms. It is important to see the irritable person behind the facade of stoicism and the domestic tyrant behind the charming personality presented in society. Should you have opportunity to observe the *Nux vomica* patient in his domestic setting in the morning and then meet him again at night, over 'wine, women and song', you will find it difficult to reconcile the two images. A *Sepia* girl — indifferent, withdrawn, sad — will suddenly thaw when she is dancing; again two apparently quite different people. The totality of symptoms will point to the appropriate drug. The totality includes both physical and mental symptoms. In a case of psychosis, for instance, the mental symptoms considered on their own will provide the diagnostic label for the condition, i.e. they are pathognomic. The concomitant physical symptoms make it possible to differentiate in cases where the disorder has onesidedly affected the mental sphere.

Hahnemann (*Organon* § 218) advises careful determination of physical symptoms present *prior* to the onset of mental illness, taking them into account in selecting the drug. This will often require help from the relatives. Such help is more easily accessible to the family doctor; 'specialists' need to make special efforts to obtain it. Holistic medicine is difficult to implement unless one knows how the individual fits into his background — of origins, family, work and environment. Knowledge of the social background enriches and deepens the patient's biography for the homoeopathic physician, giving him greater certainty in the evaluation of symptoms.

This also applies to intellectual symptoms. Intellectual capacity is the product of natural gifts and environmental factors and is markedly influenced by emotional factors. Thus perception depends on the degree of attention given to the object. Learning achievement will be poor unless there is proper motivation. This mutual determination (enhancement or depression) of emotional and intellectual functions makes it difficult to define individual contributory factors. Nature did not go to university to study psychology or the physiology of sense organs (perhaps she should have done so in this age of scientific erudition); she always presents herself as a whole. And the verbal statements made by patients usually arise out of this whole. Emotional and intellectual symptoms can often only be separated in arbitrary fashion. Kent's *Repertory* therefore lists them together under 'Mind'. Von Boenninghausen has subdivided this group of symptoms, separating off those relating to perception, thinking activity, ability to remember and freely made decisions. Dorcsi's *Symptomenverzeichnis* takes the same line, though his comments provide useful cross-references.

Summary
Symptoms relating to the emotions and intellect rank particularly high in homoeopathy. To be specific to man, medicine must base itself on what is specifically human. Anatomy and physiology relate to the animal world; emotional and intellectual contents in their specific form belong to man only.

Functional or structural changes are often preceded by those in mind and intellect. Subjective sensations make their appearance before objective changes. Prevention consists in treating changes in subjective sensation, to prevent clinical changes occurring. The drug pictures of almost all deep-acting agents include changes in mental and intellectual states. Hahnemann explored psychodynamic drug actions in his drug tests 150 years before the modern concept of psychotropic drugs evolved.

Fear and anxiety are a major element in human life. They are often only expressed indirectly. It requires skill to see behind the mask and discover the emotional suffering that lies at the back of apparently physical disorders. To the homoeopath, psychosomatic medicine is not a passing fashion. Hahnemann showed how these disorders can be treated in practice. Conversely, his *Organon* also gives guidelines for the treatment of pyschotic conditions.

Symptoms relating to the emotions and the intellect are almost always so closely bound up with each other that it is not possible to separate them in the individual case or in drug tests. Kent's *Repertory* combines them under the heading 'Mind'.

PHYSICAL SYMPTOMS

Local and General Symptoms: Patients giving their history will first of all refer to their main complaint, for it is this which has brought them to the surgery. The general inclination today is to express mental suffering in terms relating to the physical body. We must therefore learn to listen very carefully with this in mind. Depending on the kind of specialist we are, the main complaint will concentrate on a particular organ or system. Because of this, the history will initially yield mainly local symptoms. Most materia medicas and repertories give local symptoms in head-to-foot sequence. This is really quite useful if one is trying to find a particular symptom. The disadvantage for the student is that it is difficult to get the overall picture. Leeser's and Mezger's materia medicas are based on the physiology. Local symptoms will of course often give the diagnosis. Their value immediately goes up, however, if precise details are also given as to triggering factors, the nature of the symptom and its relation to time (complete symptom). They play an important part in finding the appropriate drug if they meet the conditions given in § 153 of the *Organon*. If a patient complaining of rheumatic pain says that the pain drives him from his bed at night, and he then runs cold water over his feet — this will make us prick up our ears. It is paradoxical; patients with rheumatic complaints usually need to wrap their joints up warmly. Nature does not care a fig for learned theories and biased views, however, and patients wanting cold applications need *Ledum*, *Pulsatilla*, *Guaiacum* or *Apis*. Further symptoms are needed to differentiate between these four drugs.

Differentiation depends on the totality of symptoms and we must always consider the whole person. Symptoms limited to particular localizations have to be complemented with others that involve the whole person, i.e. general symptoms.

A patient says: 'My foot hurts; I tend to feel chilly.' Or 'If I do not eat at the right time, I almost pass out from hunger. My stomach rumbles from hunger.' My almost always refers to a part; I relates to the whole person. The language tends to be very accurate. Without having to think about it, patients spontaneously tell us which are local and which general symptoms. Someone may say, perhaps beaming all over his face, 'There's nothing I like better than hard-boiled eggs' (*Calcarea carbonica*), or 'Rich foods lie heavy on my stomach' (*Pulsatilla*). Aversion from certain foods or intense desire for a particular food tell us something about the whole person, and skilful questioning is needed to differentiate symptoms in the stomach, gallbladder or intestines after certain foods from these more instinctive aversions or desires. Kent's *Repertory* lists desires and aversions under 'Stomach' and symptoms due to specific foods under the organs where they appear, e.g. 'Stomach, Pain', 'Abdomen, Pain', or 'Rectum' (constipation or diarrhoea).

Symptoms and signs of the the same kind noted in different parts of the body may be rated as general symptoms.

Example

A heavy smoker reports burning pains in his stomach. His hands and feet are icy cold, with a burning sensation as soon as they get warm. He suffers from a leg ulcer with intense burning pains from the warmth of his bed. He sticks his icy cold leg out from under the bed clothes to relieve the pain.

Each individual symptom is limited to a local area and of relatively little value. Taken together, however, the burning sensation becomes a general symptom requiring *Secale cornutum*. No other remedy has such marked burning pain with the skin icy cold, aggravated by warmth and ameliorated by cold.

There are two large groups of general symptoms which merit particular attention: **sexuality** and **sleeping habits.** Body and soul are so closely interlinked that these aspects of human life are elevated well above animal level. This in itself indicates the value which attaches to symptoms in these areas. The saying 'A quiet conscience sleeps in thunder' shows how much the quality of sleep is connected with mental factors. Most depressions come to expression in sleep disorders, with problems both in going to sleep and in sleeping through the night. Instant resort to sleeping tablets — unfortunately encouraged by many prescribers — is the most primitive of alibis for not tackling the hardest task of all — to think. Homoeopathic physicians again have a few metres head start, because they must include the more subtle elements in the history if the appropriate drug is to be found. Sleep disorders and dreams are included in the total collection of symptoms and serve as person-specific indices for particular groups of drugs.

Position during sleep is another important group including such symptoms as arms crossed under head (*Pulsatilla*); preferred side, e.g. cannot lie on left (*Phosphorus*); prefers to sleep on stomach (*Thuja, Medorrhinum*); hard pillow against small of back (*Natrum muriaticum* a.o.). Waking at certain hours of the night is indicative of certain drugs, particularly if it occurs in conjunction with specific sensations. Present-day researches into biorhythms (Forsgren) have shown that Hahnemann and his followers were excellent observers. The time relations of drug actions can in many cases be explained on the basis of peaks and troughs in our biorhythms (see Table 2). Sleeping and waking occur in a rhythm and are therefore dependent on many factors and liable to disorder. The records of homoeopathic drug tests contain many indications for sleep disorders. The repertories give time relations for individual drugs. To find the particular sleep disorder of a patient it is necessary to look under 'Sleep' and 'Modalities'. Kent's *Repertory* lists general modalities alphabetically in the section on 'Generalities'.

Dreams and frequently recurring dream sequences are a good source of material for finding the appropriate drug. The main reason for this tends to be that the interpretation of dreams takes many different forms in the various schools of psychology. Much is contradictory and transitory. Interpretation should therefore be left to those with experience. In homoeopathy, we are primarily concerned with the data obtained from drug tests. Kent's *Repertory* lists different kinds of dreams and the drugs relating to them in the section on 'Sleep' — abundant material ranging from the bright side of dreams to the soul's chamber of horrors.

Desire and love: as one would expect, there are many personal symptoms that come under this heading. If the patient does not refer to his sexual problems of his own accord, it is necessary to wait until confidence has built up. The more open the attitude on both sides — doctor and patient — the more clearly and openly are things put into words. Genuine symptoms (in the homoeopathic sense) can only be found if there is a feeling of confidence and trust. Quite a few physicians are not confided in. They are too hasty, in too much of a rush, too direct, and perhaps also unsure of themselves. The extent to which patients feel able to talk about their sexual problems is more or less a barometer indicating the atmosphere between doctor and patient. Where contact is good, sexual desires and disinclination, frigidity and impotence, premature ejaculations or the absence of orgasm will be reported. Deviations such as homosexuality, exhibitionism, nymphomania and promiscuity may also come up for discussion. It is a matter of course for the homoeopathic physician to register such things without judging them. We have no wish to sit in judgement; our aim is to help where help is asked for. Within the total picture of the patient, these symptoms belong to the deepest layer of his or her personality.

The **menstrual period** and **menstrual disorders** will be given particular attention in the case of female patients. Frequency, duration, heaviness, appearance and consistency of the menses are of importance. Pregnancy and childbirth, breast-feeding, changes or sensations in the breasts, fluor, climacteric symptoms are all important. Symptoms of this type almost always rank as general symptoms, even if they appear to be local. We should get away from merely local treatments such as dealing with bacterial and fungal infections, performing cauterizations and D&Cs, introducing local medication, irrigating and painting. We should get away from thinking in terms of replacement parts like mechanical engineers. We should look around in nature where she is still unspoilt and see and understand that marshy ground provides a habitat for marsh plants. 'It is all in the soil' (Claude Bernard). It is our job to find the homoeopathic drug which is able to change the 'soil', starting from the bottom. Psychosomatic factors involving the sexual organs, distant reactions and irritation in adjacent organs like the bladder and rectum have to be taken into account. Never forget that chronically cold feet and a chill in the lumbar region may be responsible for diseases of the pelvic organs and the bladder and kidneys. Fashionable sweaters leaving the midriff bare and blue jeans are not the right type of clothing for all seasons in our latitudes.

Summary

Physical symptoms are always considered in conjunction with observations relating to soul and spirit. We separate what basically is inseparable purely for convenience, to establish order and for ease of communication. In the same way, 'local' disease can only be understood as part of a wider context, the greater whole gives it rank and significance and also holds the potential for a cure. Listening carefully when taking the history we learn to make finer distinctions. The main complaint presented by the patient usually yields only poorly differentiated local symptoms and these are not enough to determine the appropriate drug. It is essential to have the totality of symptoms, particularly symptoms reflecting the reactivity of the whole individual and those meeting the conditions given in § 153 of the *Organon*. Characteristic and general symptoms point towards the appropriate drug. When similar sensations such as burning pains occur in different parts of the body we can follow Boenninghausen's advice and raise them to the rank of general symptoms. General symptoms are usually described by using the word 'I' — I am, I feel, I have etc. Describing local symptoms, the patient usually starts with 'my' — my knee, my arm, and so on. Desire, sleep and love are major areas yielding general symptoms. Symptoms relating to the menstrual period rank as general symptoms.

MODALITY

Homoeopathic treatment relies on accurate individualization in every single case. Without individualization it cannot succeed. We always expect tailor-made suits to be a good fit. The drug we choose should also be a good fit. It is this which makes it the simile, the appropriate homoeopathic drug. Homoeopathy can claim to be the first individualized therapy ever introduced and continues to be practically the only one to this day (excepting psychotherapy and acupuncture). It has a wider and fuller spectrum than all other therapies, encompassing the whole of body, soul and spirit. In practical terms individualization means to explore the factors connected with the onset of every sign and symptom presented by the patient. In the homoeopathic literature, these factors are referred to as 'modalities'.

Modalities establish:
— **when and due to which factors symptoms and signs are better or worse**
— **when and due to which factors symptoms and signs appear and change.**

It needs a modality or modalities to make a symptom complete. If there are no modalities we are unable to differentiate one particular drug within a group. This is something we must firmly fix in our minds. Once you know what to look for, you will find the modalities by skilful history-taking and careful observation.

The **time** is often the first modality a patient will refer to spontaneously.

Illness is a process. In the course of time it often progresses from seemingly insignificant subjective sensations to major clinical changes. The total picture also changes with time.

Two questions put to the patient when taking the history can be enormously helpful in our search for the appropriate drug:

When did these symptoms first appear?

When do you feel better or worse?

The answer to the first question will get you nowhere if the patient merely tells you the year. It is therefore advisable to amplify the question and say: 'What was going on at the time? What happened to you at that time — illness, a change of job, moving house, problems, worries?' Time of onset and aetiology complement each other to a very considerable degree, for we are not concerned with measurable time.

Modern philosophers (Jean Gebser) have shown, as have nuclear physicists (Werner Heisenberg), that time is not only quantifiable (measurable) but also has quality. In line with this, time modalities have relevance only as a measure for peaks and troughs in the life rhythms of patients. It should be remembered, however, that these rhythms are interlaced with the 'tides' of the oceans and of the earth and with the great cosmic rhythm.[4]

Answers received in response to the second question are important for homoeotherapy and its standing as a science. It is amazing how well modern research findings relating to biorhythms, Forsgren's work on the phases of liver metabolism, for instance, agree with the observations made in homoeopathic drug tests.[5]

There are also parallels to traditional Chinese medicine which gives the times of maximum and minimum energy flow within the 24-hour period of every organic region.

The 'organic clock' (Stiefvater) is important not only to acupuncturists. It is evident that when Chinese culture was at its height, the ancient physicians of that country reached a high level of achievement entirely by careful observation.

Many drug pictures have characteristic times of aggravation or change in condition within the 24-hour period that can be explained in terms of biorhythmic phases. Table 2 gives some indication of this.

Table 2: Periods of Aggravation and Biorhythms

1 a.m. *Arsenicum.*

Arsenic (a powerful capillary poison) has marked affinity to the CVS. Pain increases, anxiety, restlessness and angina, burning pains w. thirst, asthmatic symptoms w. palpitations.

Cardiovascular function is reaching its lowest point. Capillary contraction is greatest.

2 a.m. *Acidum benzoicum, Acidum nitricum.*

Ac.benzoic wakens w. anxiety, palpitations,

Renal function is at a low ebb between 2 and 3

sensation of inner heat, passing pungent urine; *Ac.nitric.* wakes up and cannot go back to sleep. Both drugs relate to uric acid diathesis, w. concentrated pungent urine.

a.m. Max. blood levels of substances due to be eliminated.

3 a.m. *Ammonium carbonicum, Kalium carbonicum, Antimonium tartaricum.* Night after night, dry cough and dyspnoea. *Kali carb.*: tormenting cough; sleepless. *Antim.tart.* coarse rattling in the chest. Cough.

At 3 a.m. the lung's vital capacity is at its lowest point, with congestion in the pulmonary circulation and venous return at a minimum.

4 a.m. *Aurum, Chelidonium, Lycopodium, Nux vomica, Podophyllum, Sulphur. Aurum* wakes up. *Chelid.* wakes into aggravation of pain and sweats. *Nux vom.* wakes with chill and cough. *Podophyl.* has abdominal pain. *Sulphur* wakes with chill.

4 a.m. is the critical period when the change-over from assimilation to dissimilation occurs. Switch-over from trophotropic to ergotropic rhythms in autonomic sphere, and to secretory functions in glandular system. All patients whose regulatory functions are out of phase and who are unable to switch easily from night-time to day-time rhythms wake up at 4 a.m.

5 a.m. *Aloe, Podophyllum, Sulphur.* The intestines react with diarrhoea at this time in all three drug pictures.

Period of maximum fat absorption in the intestinal wall has passed.

6-8 a.m. *Eupatorium, Podophyllum, Sulphur.*

Eupat. and *Pod.* feel cold. *Sulphur* is sweating. Abnormalities in heat regulation.

The body temperature begins its slow rise at this time.

9 a.m. *Carbo vegetabilis, Kalium carbonicum, Melilotus, Natrum muriaticum, Stannum.*

Carbo has haemorrhages in general, *Kali carb.* nose-bleeds when washing. *Melilot.* throbbing headache, better after nosebleed. The increased incidence of epistaxis at this hour coincides with particular painfulness of sinus conditions. *Nat.mur.* starts with general aggravation, often chills; *Stannum* has a fever.

Disorders during phase of rising temperature.

11 a.m. *Argentum nitricum, Asafoetida, Iodum, Lachesis, Natrum carbonicum, Sulphur, Zincum.*

Arg. nit. grows nervous, *Asa foet.* feels fragile, with sensation of emptiness in the epigastrium, *Iodum* is ravenous, *Lachesis* is ravenous and apt to faint, *Natrum carb.* has hunger and weakness. *Sulphur:* weak, empty, gone sensation in stomach, inclined to tears. *Zincum* has legs weak and trembling with hunger.

11 a.m. is a critical period; the dissimilatory phase in the liver is coming to an end. Blood sugar levels are often remarkably low at this time; many of the symptoms referred to are part and parcel of hypoglycaemia.

1 p.m. *Chelidonium.*
General aggravation w. burning sensation between the shoulder blades, supra-orbital neuralgia on right = neurogenic disorder relating to gallbladder.

Bile secretion is about to reach a peak.

2 p.m. *Chelidonium.*
Weak and weary, irresistible desire to sleep. Sharp pain in rt thorax and itching head.

4 p.m. *Colocynthis, Crotalus, Lycopodium, Podophyllum, Thuja.*
Colocynthis has colic w. diarrhoea, *Crotalus* heartburn. *Lycopodium* enters period of max. aggravation, w. sensation of pressure in liver.
Pod. has gastric and hepatic pain. *Thuja* enters period of aggravation, w. feeling of tightness in epigastrium.

Change-over from day to night phase in liver rhythms.

5 p.m. *Causticum, Chelidonium, China, Helleborus niger.*
Caust. and *Hell.* react w. hoarseness and cough. *China* has chilly sensation esp. in back of neck, *Hell.* cold shivers and chills.

Body temperature has reached its maximum. Circulatory output past its maximum.

6 p.m. *Argentum nitricum, Hepar sulphuris, Nux vomica, Silicea.*
All these present with cold shivers.

7 p.m. *Lycopodium, Pulsatilla, Rhus toxicodendron, Sulphur.*
Cold shivers again, or heat.   Normally body temperature going down.

9 p.m. *Aconitum, Bryonia.*
Max. temperature in cases of infection, w. fear and restlessness.

10 p.m. *Ipecacuanha, Phosphorus.*
Ip. has pseudocroup. *Phos.* apt to produce circulatory symptoms.   Circulatory output down. Minima for blood pressure and heart rate.

12 o'clock *Argentum nitricum, Lachesis.*
Fear. Cough and bouts of pain, vomiting. Oppression on chest.   Capillary contraction.

Other indicative signs and modalities will of course be needed to complement the time indications of a drug. If a patient wakes at 3 a.m., lies awake for hours, drops off to sleep again at first daylight and is irritable and cross on getting up, the sequence 'waking — sleep — waking in an irritable mood' clearly points to *Nux vomica*. If a patient reports that he could pretty well set the clock by the time the pain in his face starts again, we think of *Cedron*. Please note, it is necessary to think, to look for other signs indicative of the drug, and to write the prescription only when confirmation has been obtained.

The 'time' modality also includes other cosmic rhythms such as in spring (Kent p. 1403), in winter (Kent p. 1422), at sunrise, at full moon. Learned physicians may well smile on hearing reference made to such time-worn superstitions as the phases of the moon having an effect on people who are not well. On the other hand they have no problem with the concept of the sea rising and falling by several metres with the tides — which do relate to the phases of the moon. Phenomena are what they are, irrespective of whether they can be explained or merely (?) observed. Many phenomena relating to time can be explained on the basis of physiology, others are not open to explanation. Yet anything which helps us to find the specific drug and hence achieve a cure is of value.

Physical factors register differently even with healthy people. The sick are more sensitive — some will feel chilly if there is the slightest

Time-related Symptoms in the 24-Hour Cycle

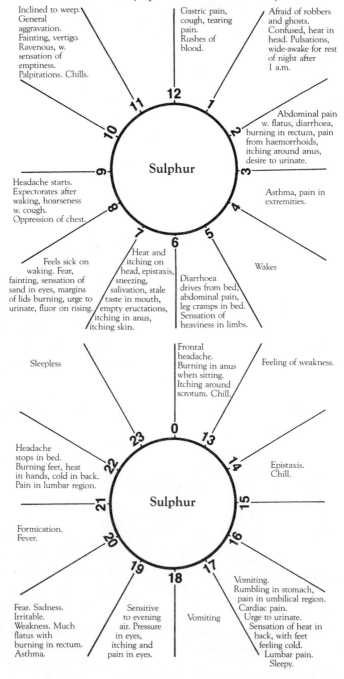

Inclined to weep.
General
aggravation.
Fainting, vertigo.
Ravenous, w.
sensation of
emptiness.
Palpitations. Chills.

Gastric pain,
cough, tearing
pain.
Rushes of
blood.

Afraid of robbers
and ghosts.
Confused, heat in
head. Pulsations,
wide-awake for rest
of night after
1 a.m.

Abdominal pain
w. flatus, diarrhoea,
burning in rectum, pain
from haemorrhoids,
itching around anus,
desire to urinate.

Sulphur

Asthma, pain in
extremities.

Headache starts.
Expectorates after
waking, hoarseness
w. cough.
Oppression of chest.

Feels sick on
waking. Fear,
fainting, sensation of
sand in eyes, margins
of lids burning, urge to
urinate, fluor on rising.

Heat and
itching on
head, epistaxis,
sneezing,
salivation, stale
taste in mouth,
empty eructations,
itching in anus,
itching skin.

Diarrhoea
drives from bed,
abdominal pain,
leg cramps in bed.
Sensation of
heaviness in limbs.

Wakes

Sleepless

Frontal
headache.
Burning in anus
when sitting.
Itching around
scrotum. Chill.

Feeling of weakness.

Headache
stops in bed.
Burning feet, heat
in hands, cold in back.
Pain in lumbar region.

Epistaxis.
Chill.

Sulphur

Formication.
Fever.

Fear. Sadness.
Irritable.
Weakness. Much
flatus with
burning in rectum.
Asthma.

Sensitive
to evening
air. Pressure
in eyes,
itching and
pain in eyes.

Vomiting

Vomiting.
Rumbling in stomach,
pain in umbilical region.
Cardiac pain.
Urge to urinate.
Sensation of heat in
back, with feet
feeling cold.
Lumbar pain.
Sleepy.

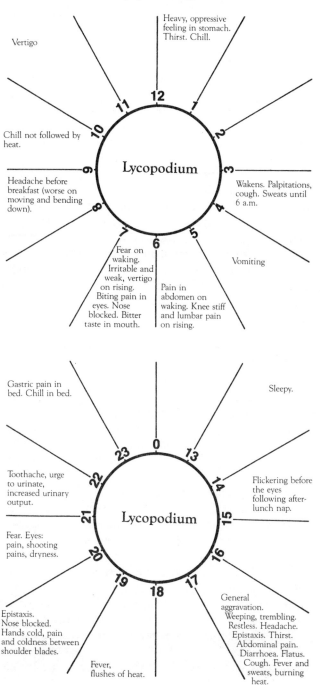

Top circle — Lycopodium

Vertigo

Heavy, oppressive feeling in stomach. Thirst. Chill.

Chill not followed by heat.

Headache before breakfast (worse on moving and bending down).

Fear on waking. Irritable and weak, vertigo on rising. Biting pain in eyes. Nose blocked. Bitter taste in mouth.

Pain in abdomen on waking. Knee stiff and lumbar pain on rising.

Wakens. Palpitations, cough. Sweats until 6 a.m.

Vomiting

Bottom circle — Lycopodium

Gastric pain in bed. Chill in bed.

Sleepy.

Toothache, urge to urinate, increased urinary output.

Flickering before the eyes following after-lunch nap.

Fear. Eyes: pain, shooting pains, dryness.

Epistaxis. Nose blocked. Hands cold, pain and coldness between shoulder blades.

Fever, flushes of heat.

General aggravation. Weeping, trembling. Restless. Headache. Epistaxis. Thirst. Abdominal pain. Diarrhoea. Flatus. Cough. Fever and sweats, burning heat.

draught (*Hepar sulphuris, Nux vomica*) others will stand by the open window and relish the icy cold air (*Iodum, Apis, Lachesis*). Some people can lie in the full sun, others 'go daft' if they do so, finding the sun hard to tolerate particularly on the head (*Glonoinum, Belladonna, Phosphorus*). There is constant guerrilla warfare in some families: Dad feels chilly and jams the windows shut (e.g. *Nux vomica*), mum is always too hot, rushes to open doors and windows, for she feels shut in if they remain closed (e.g. *Lachesis*), daughter puts on two sweaters and turns off the heating (e.g. *Pulsatilla*), son sits there in his shirt-sleeves and talks of changing the world (e.g. *Sulphur*).

Local applications must be in accord with the personal modality — if the patient is amenable. Hot packs are often helpful if there is abdominal pain (e.g. *Colocynthis*) but some patients will refuse them (e.g. *Bryonia*). Some therapists use only routine hot applications, others only cold applications. They tend to give unconscious preference to the form of application that corresponds to their own modality: *Sulphur* types are great protagonists for cold ones, *Calcarea carbonica* and *Kalium carbonicum* types for hot ones. Homoeopathic physicians need to be unbiased in considering the individual patient. It is necessary to be flexible when advising patients, for one man's meat is another man's poison.

It is no doubt healthy to sleep in an unheated room with the window open, and a cough or cold in the nose will often improve under these conditions (e.g. *Coccus cacti*). Others will get worse, however (*Bromium, Causticum, Rumex*).

Some people like to wear something on their heads even in summer (e.g. *Hepar, Silicea, Psorinum*), others go bareheaded even in the worst winter weather (*Lycopodium, Phosphorus, Iodum*).

Atmospheric conditions often have a positive or negative effect on complaints, and this is generally accepted. Something which is not generally accepted is that positive use may be made of this in choosing the appropriate drug. The modalities of weather and temperature dependence need to be enquired into particularly in chronic cases where there tends to be a paucity of individual symptoms.

One often hears of people feeling better by the sea or in the mountains, or that symptoms are worse when they are near a lake or river. These modalities have to be taken into account when making the prescription. Kent's *Repertory* lists the relevant drugs under 'Generalities' in the rubric headed 'AIR, seashore'. The rubric also applies to asthmatics, asthma being more a general than a local disease. Dorcsi lists these modalities under 'Mountain air, Sea air'.[1]

Physiological factors will give many symptoms a highly individual character. Some rheumatics feel better if completely at rest (e.g. *Bryonia*), others have to be moving (*Rhus tox.*). Most asthma patients want to sit upright in bed during an attack, perhaps bending forward with arms resting on knees (e.g. *Kalium carbonicum*) yet there are some who more or less lie on their stomachs, keeping the head low (e.g. *Medorrhinum*). Changes in position, alternation between rest and movement, stretching or bending the trunk or individual limbs all need to be enquired into, establishing their effect on the presenting symptoms.

Gastric, intestinal and renal function, the secretion of sweat, haemorrhages, sleep and sexual functions including the menses have a positive or negative effect on many symptoms. Sensory functions — vision, hearing, smell, taste, touch including sensitivity — modify a number of symptoms.

Examples
Burning gastric pain better from eating (e.g. *Graphites*), or feels better in general if constipated (*Calcarea carbonica*), or boring, screwing pain in the head worse after eating (*Calcarea phosphorica*), or headache better from passing copious amounts or urine (e.g. *Gelsemium, Kalmia*).

Mental factors will of course influence many symptoms. Some patients just have to think about their symptoms and this will make them much worse (*Acidum oxalicum*). Fear and anxiety, pleasures and sorrows, anger and annoyance influence a number of symptoms.

Examples
Vertigo in anxiety states (e.g. *Causticum*), on mental effort (*Natrum carbonicum, Natrum muriaticum, Nux vomica*); sleeplessness after good news (*Coffea*); headache after bad news (e.g. *Ignatia*).

Summary
Many different factors influence the symptoms and signs presented by the patient. The effects they produce are known as modalities. They are not rigid. Everything that is alive is in motion. Modalities arise in time and change during the time interval between preclinical and clinical condition. They are individually identified by establishing all the conditions which give rise to symptoms and signs and the time when they arise, grow worse or improve. A complete symptom covers aetiology, the nature and location of sensations, and the modalities.

SYNOPSIS OF COMMONEST MODALITIES

1   Time
    Hour, time of day, season, stage of life (infancy, childhood, adulthood, old age), onset (sudden, gradual), duration, end (rapid,

gradual), periodicity (regular recurrence — 1, 2, 7, 14 days — every spring), solar time (at sunrise, at dusk, at midnight), lunar time (full moon, new moon).

2   Physical conditions
Heat: outside temperature, room temperature, radiant heat of sun, of stove, warmth of bed, desire or disinclination to dress or wrap up warmly, head cover, dry or moist heat, temperature of bath water. Cold: outdoors, indoors. Lightly clothed, warmly dressed, draughts, dry or damp cold, pushing away bedclothes, putting out feet from under bedclothes.
Weather: before or during change in weather, change from hot to cold or cold to hot, rain, snow, wind, thunderstorms, clear or murky weather, warm, dry wind, fog.
Location: seaside, mountains, plains.
Rivers, lakes, moorland, marshy lowlands.
Basement — high-rise flat.
Indoors, outdoors, in a crowd, store, church. Narrow streets, bridges.

3   Physiological conditions
Attitude and position of body by day, at night (upright, bent; lying down, sitting, standing). Position in bed — right, left, back, arms crossed above the head, head elevated, low; prone; knee-elbow position. Rocking, tossing, turning.
Rest — movement. Walking, fast or slow; running; going up or downstairs. Travelling (train, car, plane, boat). Children allowing themselves to be carried, to be put to bed. Physical overexertion. Function of sense organs: light, noise, music, smells, taste. Response to touch — surface or deeper (desire for massage or worse from it, sensitivity to touch). Better or worse from pressure, vibration. Digestive function: food intake (solids—fluids; hunger—thirst); quantity and quality of food (little—much, hot—cold; fat—lean; sweet, sour, salty; mixing foods indiscriminately; hasty; due to certain foods. Eliminations: before, during; after stool; if constipated, with diarrhoea; on eructation, vomiting, bringing up mouthfuls of fluid, with flatus, wind.
Bladder and kidney function: before, during after urination, if little urine, a lot of urine.
Secretions: before, during, after sweat. Type of sweat. Other skin secretions. Normal and pathological secretions (tears, mucus from nose, mouth, throat, bronchi, sexual organs, anus), bleeding (normal and pathological; nose, ear, mouth, uterus, anus).
Sleep: time—duration—depth.
On going to sleep. On waking. Position.

Function of sexual organs: before—during—after menstruation, with heavy—scanty menses,
before—during—after coitus. Continence—excesses.

4   Mental factors
If thinking of illness, when experiencing fear, anxiety, pleasure, bereavement, anger, rage, fright, injured feelings, humiliation.

---

[1]   Schlueren gives some useful indications relating to gynaecology in his book. Dorcsi quite frequently refers to well-established indications in his works.

[2]   Flury R. *Homoeopathy and the Principle of Reality*, p. 57ff, establishes the philosophical and psychological reasons for the enormous value of 'sensations as if'. Both Roberts and Ward have produced good compilations of 'sensations as if'.

[3]   See Tompkins P. and Bird C. (pp. 131-5 in German edition).

[4]   This is fully discussed in Wachsmuth's *Erde und Mensch*.

[5]   With specific reference to homoeopathy, see Koehler 'Ueber die Modalität Zeit' and 'Die Zeiten der Arznei'. Ide has compiled a repertory of time modalities. I have revised his material — as yet unpublished.

[6]   Two translations of Kent's *Repertory* into German exist. Where reference is made to them in this book, the initials EK stand for Erbe Kent (publ. by Hippokrates) and KK for Keller/Kuenzli Kent (publ. by Haug).
[Reference to these is only made where the translation into German has given rise to points not evident in the original Kent and these are important in the author's presentation of a subject. Translator]

5

CASE-TAKING IN HOMOEOPATHIC PRACTICE

Case-taking in homoeopathic practice includes:

Method	Aim
Examination	Clinical diagnosis, lab. data
History-taking	Subjective data
Appearance	Establ. constitutional signs

Preconditions for good history-taking: calmness, time, patience, unbiased attitude, careful attention.

Method of history-taking: to begin with, the patient should be allowed to describe his or her complaint and sensations spontaneously; the physician then elicits further details by putting specific questions. The aim is to obtain complete symptoms (aetiology, localization, sensation, modality). To get an overall picture of the totality of symptoms, indirect questioning follows.

In cases of chronic disease, the patient's past history and family history need also be taken, to establish the constitutional background. A questionnaire saves time and is also very thorough; it will, however, depend on the individual situation and on the physician's approach and attitude whether a questionnaire is appropriate.

A patient's signs and symptoms provide the material for finding the appropriate homoeopathic drug. The significance, relative value and range of this material have been discussed in the last chapter. The next step, to be discussed in this chapter, is the encounter with the patient. It is an acquired art. There is no contradiction in saying an art has to be acquired, for both head and heart are called for in this exercise.

Encounter means that patient and physician approach each other as two equals, — no 'white-coated demigod' and 'silly, ignorant patient'. Homoeopathic case-taking can only succeed if it 'brings to light' genuine symptoms, i.e. symptoms identifying the patient as an individual. This calls for a rapport between physician and patient similar to that required in psychotherapy. If we use a simple term such as 'harmony' instead of rapport, we come really close to the aim and purpose of the encounter.

Harmony demands calm, sufficient time and patience on both sides. The patient then feels at ease and the physician is able to apply keen insight and gain an unbiased picture.

Taking the history and examining the patient will then not merely yield data but also prove therapeutic. In the encounter the homoeopathic physician gains insight into the sick person as someone who is suffering.

1 Aims

The aims of case-taking are initially the same as in modern medicine generally. A diagnosis is to be made where possible. The prognosis is determined and assessed. A treatment plan is drawn up.

In drawing up his treatment plan the homoeopathic physician decides on the basis of his skills and in all conscience whether medical homoeopathic treatment or any other form of treatment is appropriate, either on its own or in combination (surgery, diet, physiotherapy, emergency treatment, substitution, compensation, neural therapy, osteopathy, acupuncture).

If homoeotherapy is decided on, the actual job of finding the appropriate homoeopathic drug now begins.

2 Method

This aim is achieved through homoeopathic history-taking which follows on basic history-taking and extends it. Sections 83-104 in Hahnemann's *Organon* give instructions for the 'investigation and individualization of cases'. It is important to read this up in the original — and think it through. There is no better description of history-taking in the whole of the medical literature.

Some of the key ideas are the following.

Hahnemann first of all demands 'nothing but sound sense and lack of bias, careful observation and making a faithful record of the disease'. (§ 83)

Absence of bias is the first problem encountered by today's scientifically trained physician and by 'informed' patients.

The presenting symptoms are *phenomena* and we should consider them without bias or prejudice. Any thoughts of our own or interpretation will cause distortion. We must not allow ourselves to be biased by the diagnosis the patient presents with his 'collected works' (radiological reports, specialist opinions, other reports), nor should we allow our minds to fix on a particular drug which is the first to come to mind or one suggested by the evident type the patient appears to be. Clinging to a diagnosis or getting attached to a drug type are indicative of bias.

For comparison:

> A judge should never be biased. He is not allowed to pass judgement because the accused has a long record or perhaps looks like a criminal. The decision as to whether the accused is guilty or innocent rests entirely on the evidence presented by witnesses and police.

We obtain our evidence by 'careful observation' of the patient who is acting as witness in this case. It is, however, important to let the patient speak. 'He will where possible listen in silence as his patients speak, interrupting only where they run into inessentials ... Any interruption breaks the speaker's line of thought, so that afterwards they no longer remember exactly the way they were going to put things.' (*Organon* § 84).

When a condition has persisted for a long time and there are numerous symptoms it is necessary to make a record of the history (in writing or on tape), something not always necessary in acute cases, depending on one's ability to remember. 'A new line is started with every statement the patient or a member of the family makes, so that one obtains a column of individual symptoms. It is then possible to add to a symptom which initially may have been described rather vaguely but is later defined quite clearly.' (*Organon* § 85)

History-taking starts with the patient's **spontaneous report.** This covers the principal complaint, general details relating to history which point to the diagnosis, and personal symptoms. The rich variety of expression used in presenting symptoms has been discussed in the chapter on Symptomatology. Initially we do not write down anything trivial or obvious, for that would take too much time. But care is indicated, for sometimes an apparently trivial remark will later show itself to have significance, and it is essential to pay attention. We prick up our ears when something unusual, unexpected and perhaps even paradoxical crops up among the mass of common detail (think of a rheumatic patient who puts his painful feet in cold water). The patient's spontaneous report must be taken purely phenomenologically, as regards both content and the words chosen, and there should be careful attention and no prejudice. *Observe* the patient — but avoid the fixed stare of the public prosecutor. A momentary blush, a slight gesture, silence in between — these can say so much. Or else a fountain of verbosity can leave so much unsaid. The spoken word often only assumes real value if these nuances are considered. You will soon learn to distinguish between under and overstatement. The patient's presentation of the case often makes it possible even at this stage to distinguish between organic lesion, functional disorder and mental suffering.

Specific questions are asked after the spontaneous report. 'Once a speaker has said all he or she wants to say the physician adds the finer detail for every single symptom.' (*Organon* § 86). Ideally such 'finer detail' leads to a complete symptom (see Chapter 4, 4, p. 45), though it cannot be forced. Section 87 has the following warning:

> The physician then asks for finer detail relating to every statement made by the patient, taking care not to put leading questions or questions requiring only yes or no for an answer; this could induce the patient to confirm or deny something that is not true, or only a half-truth, or else does indeed apply — taking the line of least resistance or wishing to please. The inevitable result is the wrong picture of the disease and the wrong form of treatment.

Added comment: 'The physician must not ask, for instance, whether a particular circumstance did or did not pertain. No physician should ever be guilty of making such suggestions, which must lead to the wrong answer and statement.'

Nevertheless our goal, the complete symptom, must be achieved.

Consistently and with due caution the answers have to be found to the following questions:

Cur? — Why? Due to what? Triggering factor?
Aetiology
e.g. injury, chill, annoyance, dietary indiscretion.
Ubi? — Where?
Location of signs, of pain.
Quod? — What? How?
Nature of signs and symptoms, of sensations, of pain
e.g. ulceration of mucosa with burning pain.
Quomodo? — When? Factors causing aggravation or amelioration?
Time and/or *factor* relating to improvement or worsening of symptoms and signs
e.g. pain worse due to cold wind.

Repeated negative experience — not only with students — forces me to repeat most emphatically that in many cases the appropriate remedy can only be found on the basis of *complete symptoms*.

The questions have not been put in Latin to sound academic, but because this helps us to remember — two with *u*, two with *o*:

Cur   Ubi
Quod   Quomodo

Indirect Questions: a history based on spontaneous report and specific questions is usually adequate in acute and entirely local conditions.

It is not adequate for protracted chronic conditions. The *totality of symptoms* will be needed. The patient cannot know how curious the species *Medicus homoeopathicus* is, i.e. what kind of information he needs, and questions must therefore be put.

> If several parts or functions of the body have not been mentioned in this voluntary report, the physician will ask what else comes to mind with reference to those parts and functions, and also concerning the patient's state of mind, but in general terms, so that the speaker is forced to use his or her own specific words. (*Organon* § 88)

Hahnemann again reminds us that suggestion must be avoided; we are to put our questions 'in general terms'.

The sequence in which questions are put will depend on personal taste and the given situation. Every physician should evolve his or her own basic system and keep this well in mind. It is easy to forget things in the course of conversation that may nevertheless be important. A clear system provides a good basis for individual variation, for individualization also applies in this case.

For practical reasons it is advisable to inquire into individual organs in head-to-foot sequence. Most repertories and materia medicas follow this system.

Next come the general symptoms. These convey an impression of overall reactivity. They include modalities affecting the whole person. Local and general modalities may be contradictory, e.g. *Arsenicum* patients tend to be chilly but like coolness to the head.

Questions as to the state of mind come last, though they are the most important. But there's no point in springing this on people. Much can already be deduced from the basic symptomatology and observation of the patient when history-taking. Enquiries into the state of mind call for 'particular circumspection, thoughtfulness, knowledge of human nature, gentleness in one's probing, and patience to a high degree' (*Organon* § 98). Again direct questions must be avoided, for they provoke untruthfulness. Ask ten men if they are afraid. I'll bet eight will reply in the negative. Approach the issue indirectly therefore, using examples like: 'Even some adults feel ill at ease in the dark (or in a thunderstorm, up a steep slope, with dogs, with large animals etc.); have you ever noticed anything like this?' Or: 'Sometimes a person feels they'd like to put an end to their life — would you be able to understand this?' Or: 'I went to a concert the other day. The woman sitting next to me started to weep silently. I suppose the music did rather go to the heart . . . ?' You will immediately get a positive or negative response to this kind of indirect question. (*Natrum carbonicum, Natrum sulphuricum, Graphites* and a few other drugs have this symptom — Kent p. 94.)

It should also be remembered that 'mind' symptoms may vary considerably in the course of the day or with the seasons. Many people are depressed in the mornings but lively at night (e.g. *Lachesis*), something to be remembered when someone seems 'full of beans' at evening surgery. One should perhaps say to such a person: 'We have had a most stimulating talk now; how do you see things in the early morning?' Or: 'Now that it is winter you have few problems with your nerves, as you have told me. Of course some people don't feel quite so good in spring or in summer . . .?

Dishonourable or embarrassing episodes, suicide attempts, profound mortification from unhappy or painful memories, jealousy, rage, hatred, envy, avarice, pride, destructive impulses will only be elicited by a 'happy turn of phrase in putting the question' (footnote to *Organon* § 93). Drug addicts, alcoholics and syphilitics are almost all liars. Listen to the misrepresentations, never displaying the missionary zeal of one laying sole claim to the truth. If possible, watch the eyes and the mouth of the speaker at one and the same time. No one is able to keep control over both at the same time. Unconscious elements will overlay conscious ones.

> Every physician should study physiognomy and be able to interpret its signs in sickness and in health. Before we send a patient for an X-ray we should look at him or her. Sophisticated instruments must not be allowed to block our view of the individual person. There is a time for everything — first look, then use the penetration of X-rays. One sometimes wonders which will give the more profound insight. Personally I have found Huter's physiognomy of great value.[1]

Everything a patient says should in principle be taken for true. Unreasonable expectations and prejudices have to be suppressed. Even exaggerated reports should be taken for truth.

> Pure invention of incidentals and complaints is unlikely even in the case of hypochondriacs, including the most insufferable . . . It is, however, necessary to deduct a little from those exaggerated statements and ascribe at least the powerful form of expression to an excess of feeling; in this respect even the high pitch of expression in describing their suffering becomes one more significant symptom among those making up the picture of the disease. It is another matter with people of unsound mind and malicious inventors of illness. (Part of footnote to *Organon* § 96)

'Malicious inventors of illness' are rare. They always have a motive and this can often be discerned: to gain power through illness. The modern welfare state provides a cushy life for quite a few parasites; and there are those who are experts in this field. The homoeopathic materia medica has something to offer even for this kind of mentality. It is to be regretted that the rubrics Work, aversion to mental, Indolence and Dullness (Kent pp. 95, 55 and 37) are thirty times the length of Industrious (Kent p. 56). A philosopher might conclude that indolence is the norm.

Man is a sociable animal. Assessment of 'mind' symptoms must include the person's position and attitude in the nuclear and wider family, nation, state, world of work and all other social contexts. These are not normally referred to in the spontaneous report and observation and indirect questions will have to provide the necessary information in this area. The sick person as someone playing an active role in life will show his individuality in excessive demands (e.g. cannot bear to be left alone) or extreme denial (e.g. refuses to be spoken to — Kent p. 82). Certain aspects of human contact behaviour may already be observed in the waiting room and then on greeting the patient, from gestures and speech. The difference in readiness to make contact between introverts (often thin, chilly, pale individuals) and extraverts (often large, warm, red people) must be taken into consideration as typological background for all individual variations. Those variations will only have symptomatic value if they go beyond a certain limit of tolerance. Intensity and differences between then and now make typological differences into valuable symptoms: misanthropy, fear of people, antipathy towards marriage partners, own children, hatred, murderous instincts (Desire to kill — Kent p. 60).

The spontaneous report, specific questions and indirect questions yield a good cross-section of the present condition.

BIOGRAPHY

The final point of interest is the longitudinal section provided by biography. What heredity, constitutional weaknesses, morbid factors created the 'soil' which causes this particular person to suffer from this particular disease? Information is obtained through family history, personal history of previous illnesses, treatments (suppression?), vaccinations. Further data arise from an evaluation of the totality of symptoms.

I have deliberately saved the biography for the end of this chapter, although it is usual to start with the family and personal histories. Unfortunately they tend to be given short shrift, perhaps even just the terse comment: previous history negative.

Homoeopathy makes use of phenomena both past and present in the search for the appropriate drug. In cases of chronic disease, symptoms preceding the present status are often important. A clinical, pathological lesion is the end product of a long process in which pathogenetic factors confronted autonomic regulation and the self-healing potential of the organism. To achieve a cure we need personal symptoms rather than symptoms obviously arising from the sheer mechanics of an anatomical lesion (e.g. by occupying space). Few personal symptoms remain when the final, burnt-out stage has been reached. If there is to be any hope beyond merely palliative relief using organotropic drugs, symptoms which came earlier in time need to be taken into account. We need valuable general and 'mind' symptoms and their modalities. This explains the great significance attaching to the previous history in homoeopathic case-taking.

SUGGESTIONS FOR INDIRECT QUESTIONS
First area to be enquired into: Local symptoms in head to foot sequence:

Head
    Hair, complexion, eyes, nose, mouth, oral cavity, teeth, tongue, tonsils
    Sensory functions: vision, hearing, smell, taste
    Headache
Throat
    Outside — inside
    Larynx — voice — goitre
    Trachea
Chest
    Thorax
    Heart
    Breast
    Oesophagus
Lung
    Respiration
    Bronchi
    Cough
Abdomen
    Stomach, gastric pain, eructations, heartburn
    Intolerance of foods (for dislike of foods, see General symptoms)
    Abdomen
    Rectum, stools
Back
    Back of neck, spine

Extremities
  Shoulder, arms, hip, legs
Bladder — kidneys
  Inflammation, continence, pain
  Urination
Genitalia
  Penis, testes, prostate, discharges
  Vulva, uterus, ovary, fluor.

Second area to be enquired into: General symptoms concerning the whole person

Food and fluid intake
  Appetite
  Desire for or dislike of certain foods or drinks
Water metabolism
  Thirst
  Sweat
  Oedema
Sleep
  Sleeplessness
  Depth of sleep
  Restfulness of sleep
  Sleeping position
  Dreams
Skin
  Inflammation, eruption, warts, scars, marks, tumours
Vertigo
Modalities affecting the whole person (see Chapter 4)
  Time, hour, season, sun, moon
  Physical conditions: heat, cold, weather, locality
  Physiological conditions: position, posture, lying down, rest,
    movement
  Function of sense organs: light, noise, smells, sensations to
    touch
  Elimination: secretions, excretions
Mind and intellect
  Intellect, memory
  Temper: equable, exalted, cheerful, sad
  Anger, rage, hatred, envy, avarice, pride
  Destructive impulses towards things, people, oneself
  Attitude to praise, words of comfort
  Fear, anxiety, things imagined, delusions

Sexual functions and sexuality
    Desire, aversion, neutral
    Potency, orgasm, deviation from normal drives
    Menses: cycle, duration, amount, colour, consistency
    Changes in well-being before, during, after menses
    Pain
    Births, breast-feeding

Third area to be enquired into: Longitudinal section through pathogenesis — medical biography

Family
    Illnesses and predisposition of parents and siblings
    Causes of death, hereditary diseases
    Childhood illnesses, childhood experiences, disappointments, shock etc.
    Later illnesses, treatments, medication received
    Suppressive therapy, vaccinations
    Operations, traumas
Predisposition
    Constitution
    Diathesis
    Strokes of fate, losses, humiliation, injured feelings
    Occupation, stresses at work, job satisfaction
Attitude to environment
    Parents, siblings, husband, wife, children, other people

3 Using a Questionnaire in Case-Taking

Taking the case-history personally is time-consuming, but one also sees, hears, smells and encounters the whole person. It is indeed the 'imponderables' which lend colour to the picture. All our sense organs are live antennae; they reinforce or reduce the significance of what the patient is saying.

'The physician sees, hears, perceives with his other senses what has changed or is unusual in these.' (*Organon* § 84) Nevertheless a questionnaire can be useful, for it saves time. I think it will depend on the particular patient and on the physician whether the history is taken personally or with the aid of a questionnaire. Physicians more inclined to 'sense' things will have little use for a questionnaire. They need to experience the living play of movement in the patient to give them ideas. Physicians who are more 'word orientated' find it easier to spot the principal signs with the aid of a questionnaire. The to and fro of speech, gesture, movement and dialogue tends to confuse and distract in their case. To say this implies no judgement of any kind.

Questionnaires have been designed by Kent, Eichelberger and Voegeli among others. All have their advantages and their limits. It is obvious that patients asked to fill in such a questionnaire must be reasonably intelligent, co-operative and interested in the truth.

4 Time Expended on Case-Taking

Time needs to be saved in any kind of practice nowadays. Experienced physicians will be able to work more quickly than beginners, and the situation is different in every case, so that it is not possible to lay down a time limit in advance. If an appointment system is in operation, half or three quarters of an hour will have to be allowed for a first appointment for someone with a chronic condition. More than that is too much for both doctor and patient. It is better to make another appointment for the clarification of further points. Twenty minutes are usually sufficient for a second appointment.

Summary

Good case-taking provides a complete cross and longitudinal section of the current illness and its genesis. 'Once the totality of the symptoms which predominantly determine and distinguish the case has been accurately recorded, or in other words one has obtained the picture of the disease in a particular case, the hardest part of the work has been done.' (*Organon* § 104)

Case-taking will only be successful if the relationship between doctor and patient is harmonious. Calmness, time and patience are major preconditions if rapport is to be established. In this way history-taking and examination are a form of stock-taking and as such already therapeutic. A homoeopathic physician uses a double approach: examination and history-taking follow the lines laid down in medical school and clinical teaching. They establish the pathological diagnosis and the prognosis, and lead to a plan of treatment. The latter encompasses the decision as to whether medical, homoeopathic or other — e.g. surgical — treatment is indicated.

If the decision is in favour of homoeopathic treatment, homoeopathic history-taking follows. Its sole aim is to find the particular drug appropriate to the case.

This dual approach does require more time and greater personal commitment, none of which is taken into account in schedules of fees. A physician deciding for homoeotherapy will gain in job satisfaction and have the pleasure of a happy outcome even in apparently hopeless cases. It is a matter of personal choice.

Sections 83-104 of the *Organon* give a classic description of homoeopathic history-taking. This calls for lack of bias, careful attention and a faithful record of the disease picture. Homoeopathic case-taking proceeds in three stages:

1 Spontaneous report: only the patient speaks.
2 Specific questions: doctor and patient work together to add missing detail to the spontaneous report. These two stages are normally all that is needed in acute cases. Chronic cases also call for
3 Indirect questions: to get the totality of symptoms. All the areas the patient has not touched on are now considered. Indirect questioning means that all suggestion must be avoided.

The type of indirect question put will depend on the situation. It is best to have a definite system of one's own and keep this well in mind. One suggestion — in line with the system used in most repertories and materia medicas — is:

1 local symptoms on the head-to-foot system
2 general symptoms
3 modalities relating to the whole person
4 mind symptoms
5 sexual symptoms.

Such triple 'cross-questioning' will almost always yield complete and personal symptoms. These usually include quite a few biographical details.

The medical biography comprising family history and past history of the patient completes the longitudinal section. Evaluation of the symptoms permits their classification in constitutional terms, in accord with Hahnemann's view of chronic disease.

A well-designed questionnaire can aid history-taking. It will be based on more or less the same system as personal case-taking. Physicians very much in the habit of using their eyes will find it difficult to perceive the principal signs when reading through a completed questionnaire. Those more theoretically inclined on the other hand may find it better to use a questionnaire rather than the very personal atmosphere of taking the history oneself, the latter being more likely to confuse and distract. The patient needs to contribute intelligence, co-operation and a desire for truthfulness.

In practice, the encounter and dialogue with the patient will never be as schematic as this. Yet it is necessary to have a basic structure. It will then be possible in the individual case to use clear judgement and make both rapid and effective assessment. The aim is to save time and yet have optimum quality. Efficiency in determining the appropriate drug depends solely and entirely on the quality of case-taking. Once this has been done, the homoeopathic physician has the hardest part of the job behind him.

Below, three examples are given where 'cough' was the main complaint, the aim being to put life into the theoretical foundations. The dialogue was put down in writing shortly after taking the history in each case. It has been based on the notes taken of the history. It might have been even better to record the history on tape for this purpose.

Examples

1 Mr W. K., pensioner, age 66 years
Appearance: Pallid, yellowy face. Slim. Posture slack. Hands cold (noted when shaking hands).
Main complaint: Cough for 6 weeks, with blood-stained mucus during last week. No pain.
On examination the tongue was moist, greyish white, tonsils atrophic. Nasal breathing free, watery coryza (always examine nasopharynx if there is a cough). Voice husky, rough. Bronchitic sounds much in evidence over lung base, no dullness. Laryngoscopy not possible because of retching reflex. Varicosities at back of pharynx. Liver enlarged by two fingers. Fatty liver diagnosed at an earlier date. Smokes a lot. ESR normal, hepatic enzymes greatly elevated. Differential diagnosis: bronchogenic carcinoma? carcinoma of larynx? cirrhosis of the liver? smoker's bronchitis? bronchiectases?
Treatment plan: referred to ENT for full diagnosis.
Subsequent report: operable carcinoma of the larynx. No homoeopathic therapy initially. This also obviated the need for further history-taking.

2 Mrs W. Ch., clerk in commercial firm, age 52 years. Widow, one son aged 28.
Appearance: dark-haired, vivacious lady using expressive gestures, dark complexion.
Main complaint: 'Always coughing'.
On examination nasopharynx n.a.d., lung n.a.d., routine X-ray 3 months earlier n.a.d. Diagnosis: cough syndrome of uncertain origin.
Spontaneous report: 'The cough drives me crazy — it's been going on for years — sometimes it is better, sometimes worse. Oh yes, the more I let it upset me the worse the cough gets. And always my mouth feels sticky inside, so dry my tongue sticks to the roof. I think the cough comes from my stomach — the air pushes upwards. Then I sometimes feel as if I would faint. My boss wants the work done quickly — I can't keep up any more. I keep forgetting things, names and so on — sometimes I feel quite numb — then I have to cough again.'

Specific questions:
Doctor: 'You said the cough has persisted for some years. Do you recall

in any way when all this coughing started? Was there anything special in your life at the time?'

Patient: 'Not at the time, or maybe yes; I had got terribly upset. It's something like six years ago. I could not talk for coughing, I could not get any air. I collapsed, my son put me on the couch. Suddenly he was really concerned about me. Oh no, he is always touchingly concerned, but at that time, when he met the girl who is now his wife, his mother did not exist, she was practically forgotten.'

Doctor: 'Have you noticed anything else, anything other than nervous excitement, that will make the cough worse? Some people will only cough when it is raining, others if the atmosphere is dry. What affects you most?

Patient: 'You know, in the autumn when it gets foggy, I want to creep into my shell like a snail; cold, wet weather is poison to me. Then the stupid cough never stops. And if then my daughter-in-law comes in and starts talking of Christmas already, my hands go icy cold and I cough. It simply upsets me, but young people, what do they know!'

Doctor: 'You said your mouth often feels dry. What do you do about it?'

Patient: 'Nothing really. I do not like to drink much, it only fills up my stomach even more. A mint perhaps, but it does not help much.'

Doctor: 'When your stomach is that full, what comes up, air or fluid?'

Patient: 'Just air mostly. It feels really good. I find it embarrassing to have so much wind, but it does relieve it.'

Doctor: 'You said you sometimes felt as though you would faint.'

Patient: 'Yes, I almost pass out.'

Doctor: 'On what kind of occasion?'

Patient: 'Oh, when I get upset, it really pulls the legs from under me. I go quite numb, everything seems far away, my boss behind his desk is miles away.'

Doctor: 'What kind of things do you forget?'

Patient: 'Everything often. My head is a balloon then and simply cannot think.'

Doctor: 'Balloon?'

Patient: 'My head feels large, and I can feel my heart beating.'

Doctor: 'How is your heart beating?'

Patient: 'Hard, in my head and also in my body.'

Indirect questions:

Doctor: 'You have told me quite a lot already, but perhaps we should also consider how you are otherwise. Do you have any other sensations in the head?'

Patient: 'In the head — a headache sometimes, specially when I have been drinking alcohol. I simply can't take alcohol any more. In the old days, when my husband was still alive, I quite liked a drink occasionally.'

Local symptoms were then enquired into, following the head-to-foot system. Nothing really new was said about eyes, ears, mouth, lungs. Under 'Desire for and dislike of certain foods — intolerance of foods' she said that she liked well-seasoned foods. 'Anything without much flavour tastes like cardboard to me', but tolerated all foods well if equanimous as far as her nerves were concerned. If upset — and she often was upset — epigastric fullness developed rapidly even after a light meal and she felt sick, got the hiccups and grew hypersensitive to anything with a relatively strong smell. Stools generally good. But sometimes she had to push quite hard and had a feeling as if she was constipated. It then seemed all the more surprising to her that the stools were soft after all. 'It won't come out; it really is the limit. I have got to stay on the toilet for a while then, otherwise I'll simply pass out.'

Her periods tended to be rather variable in the past. They usually lasted 6 days, with very dark menses from the second day onwards. Periods stopped 6 years ago.

As to her state of mind, she said: 'I often do not understand myself. My son says 'You're like an April day, with rain soon followed by sunshine.' It is true, I will easily feel sad and then just as quickly be laughing again. After all that has happened in my life I am glad I can cheer up quickly.'

Evaluation: the history is rather mixed, but even the spontaneous report ('my cough is driving me mad') indicated that the condition was unlikely to be specifically limited to the nasopharynx or pulmonary system. Examination confirmed this. A physician geared only to organic pathology would have to throw in the towel at this point. After all, what could he do in this case? It is quite impossible to attach a diagnostic label to the condition and therefore to have a basis for treatment in organic pathology.

The homoeopath finds this a fascinating history. Let us first of all look for peculiar and characteristic symptoms in the spontaneous report:

1   The more I get upset the more do I cough.
2   Sticky, dry feeling in mouth, tongue sticks to the roof. Paradoxically the tongue is moist on examination.
3   Feels numbed, as though about to faint, forgetful.
4   Cough coming from stomach, air pushing upwards.

Specific questioning yielded further material, the aim being to get symptoms that are as complete as possible.

Aetiology: started after an upset 6 years ago, when her son became less attentive.

Sensation: dry cough, no pain.

Modality: started with and worse on getting upset, worse in cold wet weather.

Concomitants:

i)   Sensation of dryness in mouth, tongue sticks to roof, but no thirst ('I do not like to drink a lot').
ii) Fullness in stomach, with eructation of air which relieves. Cough coming from stomach.

Other symptoms, not directly related to the cough which is the main complaint:

a)   Sensation of faintness and fullness of stomach, if upset, after passing stools; concomitant symptom: everything recedes, 'as if boss were miles away'. Interpretation of this symptom: objects surrounding one appear smaller when feeling faint.

The head, on the other hand, is felt to be enlarged (balloon), 'I can feel my heart beating in my head.'

b) Indirect questioning yielded a peculiar symptom relating to stools: feels as if constipated, stools do not pass easily, although soft; feels faint after passing stools.

c) Periods (in the past) variable, prolonged dark blood.

d) State of mind 'like April day', mood changes quickly, now cheerful, now sad, for no adequate reason.

Comment: the totality of symptoms in this case corresponded to the drug picture of *Nux moschata*. This drug cured her 'nervous cough', dry mouth, attacks of faintness, eructation of air, abdominal fullness and problems with stools. The relationship with her daughter-in-law improved. Her forgetfulness at work was less of a problem to her. Variations in mood persisted, at least for the period of observation.

NB: We will hardly be able to change a person's basic nature, for experience has shown that this is something we are born with and which determines our life.

Anyone familiar with the drug picture of *Nux moschata* will quickly spot the similarity. The drug shows a characteristic 'inclination to react hysterically' with eructation of air for no apparent reason, dryness of mouth but no thirst, stools difficult to pass although soft.

3   R.Sch., a schoolboy 10 years of age

Appearance: light-skinned, ashblond, fidgety, won't sit still. Has been brought by his mother who gives most of the history herself.

Main complaint: has been previously treated for severe colds; this time violent cough and shortness of breath for 1 week.

On examination a 'snotty nose' was found. Nose blocked, whitish mucus in pharynx, tonsils slightly enlarged, no inflammation. Plenty of moist rales all over lung, also rhonchi and wheezes, particularly on expiration.

Pathological diagnosis: caterrhal infection with asthmatoid bronchitis.

Spontaneous report: 'He must have caught a cold when we went for quite a long ramble in the Black Forest last Sunday. He keeps the whole family awake at night with his barking cough, and he is also wheezing. For the last 2 days he has also been short of breath and gasping for air just like his uncle who has had asthma for a long time.'

Specific questions:

Doctor: 'The weather was pretty rotten last Sunday — we went on a ramble as well and at the top we found ourselves in clouds of fine rain.'

Mother: 'Yes, he was dressed warmly, but he will keep on talking and run this way and that, so his feet were wet when we got home at night.'

Doctor: 'How long has he had this cough?'

Mother: 'His nose was running the next day, but he only started barking on Monday night.'

Doctor: 'Rolf — it sometimes hurts when one has a cough.'

Rolf: 'Not me, only I can't run so well.'

Mother: 'Yes, he has to stop quite a lot.'

Doctor: 'What comes out when you cough?'

Mother: 'Nothing, I think, he swallows everything down, I keep telling him . . .'

Doctor: 'You say he is coughing at night, when does it start, immediately on going to bed or later?'

Mother: 'It really gets worse later on, I think it must be after midnight and more towards morning.'

Doctor: 'When is he so short of breath, then?'

Mother: 'When he's running around, and also at night.'

Doctor: 'Does he get up then?'

Mother: 'Sometimes, but he coughs even more when he goes to the toilet.'

Doctor: 'How does he lie in his bed?'

Mother: 'Ah yes, that is something I have noticed. I had put several pillows to his back. Uncle thought he'd find it easier to breathe that way, sitting up (he suffers from asthma). But Rolf had thrown all the pillows out and towards morning, when I looked in, he was lying flat on his stomach, and his head had slipped down quite low to the edge of the bed. He was sleeping quietly and also breathing quite regularly.'

Doctor: 'Does he often sleep on his stomach?'

Mother: 'Yes, sometimes on his back, but I often find him sleeping on his stomach. They say that is good for children.'

Doctor: 'Is there anything else you have noticed?'

Mother: 'Well, you know how fidgety he is, his teacher is always complaining. He says the boy lacks concentration and that is why he keeps making mistakes and forgets things so quickly.'

Doctor: 'He's a bright lad, isn't he? What is harder, arithmetic or spelling?'

Mother: 'He does quite well in arithmetic, if he wants to. But he will make the daftest mistakes in spelling.'

Doctor: 'Anything else — his head, his stomach, the skin, arms or legs?'

Mother: 'Mainly his cough. I hope he won't get asthma, like his uncle, I really dread this. Will he need to have a little pump as well?'

Doctor: 'One more question, I think. When he is short of breath, do you have the feeling that he gets anxious about it? It could be.'

Mother: 'How about it, Rolf?'

Rolf: 'Och, I simply stop running.'

Doctor: 'You went to the North Sea coast last year. How did he do there?'

Mother: 'It was super at the seaside. He had still been coughing at home, but up there it had all gone in no time.'

Indirect questions yield nothing of particular value.

Evaluation: a boy of 10 inclined to catch colds develops asthmatoid bronchitis after exposure to cold, damp weather. Asthma is present in the family (mother's uncle). The spontaneous report provides no further symptoms. With children it is often necessary to rely on visible signs and the details given by parents. The boy's fidgety restlessness is obvious; he walks about in the consulting room. Specific questions elicit that the cough at night occurs more after midnight and towards morning. The cough is painless, expectoration minimal and cannot be assessed. Dyspnoea worse on running about and after prolonged bouts of coughing. The position in sleep is striking: he wants to lie flat on his stomach with the head low and then coughs less and has no dyspnoea — quite the opposite of the uncle who sits upright propped against a mound of bedding. Asthmatics lying that low are a rarity. The boy is not anxious when dyspnoeic. A seaside holiday was good for him, he did not cough whilst there.

Further symptoms: the fidgetiness which was immediately apparent caused problems at school. Oddly enough he concentrates less well when writing than when doing arithmetic.

Summing up:

Aetiology: from cold, wet weather.

Sensation: cough, no pain; dyspnoea.

Modality: cough worse after midnight, towards morning. Dyspnoea worse on running, after much coughing. No anxiety. Better in prone position, with head low.

Further symptoms: lacks concentration, fidgety, won't sit still. At school good at sums, frequent spelling errors.

Comment: The totality of symptoms corresponds to the drug picture of *Medorrhinum*. The principal symptom is: cough and dyspnoea better when prone, worse from cold, wet weather. Fidgety, lacking in concentration, forgetful, poor spelling.

[1] For literature, apply to Carl Huters Werke, Siegfried Kupfer, Schwaig b. Nuremberg, FRG.

6

DIFFERENT METHODS OF DETERMINING THE APPROPRIATE DRUG (DRUG DIAGNOSIS)

A number of different methods may be used to find the appropriate drug in a case.

The conditions pertaining in medical practice often force us to make rapid decisions and save time. These are the 'short cuts' to drug diagnosis. It should always be remembered, however, that time-saving methods must also give reliable results.

Where this is not possible because of the situation of patient or physician, the 'long road' will have to be taken, establishing the totality of symptoms by careful individualization. Evaluation can be difficult if there are too few or too many symptoms (patient too lazy to talk or else talkative).

Many of the mistakes made in choosing the drug are avoidable. The principal fault usually lies in ourselves, being a lack of self-criticism. Every physician is free to choose the method best suited to him or her and to the given situation, taking into account his or her knowledge of materia medica and personal inclinations.

Physicians may be inclined to be analytical or to think more in terms of synthesis. These are different but equally valid approaches.

1 Preconditions for Reliable Results
Quality of Case-Taking
The last two examples given in the chapter on homoeopathic case-taking touched on the heart of the matter where finding the appropriate drug is concerned. The personal distinguishing symptoms and signs of the patient guide us in the search for the homoeopathic, i.e. 'similar', drug. An abstract collective label attached to the disease will open no doors for us. The sick individual person is the standard. Symptoms and signs are the mirror image in which we perceive similarity to the drug. Case-taking and drug diagnosis thus merge into one another in so far as phenomenological comparison is made to establish similarity.

The drug diagnosis will show if we have grasped the patient as a person, as a unique individual, in our case-taking; it will show whether we heard 'where the shoe pinches'; whether we have perceived the patient's illness as a process, a life story. This may be the point where it becomes obvious that we have merely been collecting obvious diagnostic labels, that the symptoms we have recorded are too general and colourless; that we have not got a single complete symptom. Reliability of drug diagnosis depends on the quality of case-taking. Hahnemann gives encouragement when he says that once the case has been taken, 'the hardest part of the work has been done' (*Organon* § 104). When a hard task has been done it is good to take a break. A break in which to think things over. It is advisable to distance oneself to some extent so as to get a clear overview of the material gained on case-taking before we rush to consider individual symptoms in our eagerness. It is best to gain an overview before getting lost in detail.

A CLEAR IMAGE OF THE DISEASE
Section 3 of the *Organon* demands that we aim to get a clear image of the disease. No mention is made as yet of symptoms, though generally speaking the patient's symptoms dominate the picture. Here, at the very beginning of his *Organon*, Hahnemann wrote: 'If the physician clearly perceives what morbid conditions are present, where healing is specifically needed in every individual case (perception of morbid state, indication) . . ., he will know how to take efficient and effective action.'

Voisin probably gave the best definition of this process when he said: 'We have to grasp the nature of the disorder.' Eichelberger has referred to the 'idea inherent in a case of illness.'

Once we have grasped the nature of a disorder, the idea inherent in a case of illness or the morbid condition, the symptoms and their modalities really come to life and assume significance in drug diagnosis. Please note: perception of the illness is not the same as knowing the name of the disease or its nosological classification. Perception of the illness has to do with the answer to the question: Why has this patient contracted this particular illness at this stage? It aims to grasp the disorder in the patient. What happened to this person? Was it some external factor, physical trauma? Have his feelings been injured, has he experienced trouble, sorrow, worries, a stroke of fate? Or will we be able to understand his symptoms if we consider his constitution, the inherited or acquired diathesis? And the final question, unfortunately one of increasing relevance in the present age: Could the patient's symptoms and signs be due to treatment received, to the medical or surgical 'suppression' of physiological or pathological discharges? Or to drug damage? Have those factors caused pathophysiological or morphological changes which may explain the clinical picture?

To get a clear image of the disease we must first of all consider the aetiology of the disorder.

It will always be necessary to consider how far examination of the patient covers the major points of differential diagnosis. Perceiving the illness also means evolving a treatment plan in which the 'efficient and effective' (*Organon* § 3) sequence of therapeutic measures and use of adjuvant measures (diet, life-style) are considered.

The material obtained on case-taking is not normally homogeneous; its tends to be multi-layered.

Example
A female patient comes to the surgery on account of migraine persisting for 10 years. When case-taking had been concluded and she was almost on the door-step, taking her departure, she mentioned, embarrassed and with some hesitation, that she had sprained her knee 2 weeks earlier whilst skiing. She had been to see an orthopaedic surgeon who had applied ointment and a dressing to the knee. The pain was better, but she now had a burning, itching eruption on the knee.

Inspection: red vesicular eruption, joint slightly swollen, minor limitation of movement.

Diagnosis: contact eczema, post-strain status.

The aetiology of the acute disorder and the appearance of the skin agree with the drug picture of *Rhus toxicodendron*. It is logical to consider the acute situation first in this case, only considering the migraine symptoms after this in choosing the appropriate drug.

It is necessary to establish whether the acute state is a flare-up of the constitutional disorder or is of extraneous origin — like the sprain and the contact eczema in this case.

To perceive the real illness also requires a good deal of self knowledge. The physician must ask himself or herself: What can I do in this case, what do I know with certainty concerning the patient and the drug needed in this case? More generally, we must ask: Where do my particular gifts lie? Do I see more clearly or hear more clearly? Am I more analytical or synthetic in my thinking? What is the real nature of the particular case in which a decision has now to be made? Do the things I have learned from the patient match a drug picture I am familiar with?

Case-taking and finding the appropriate drug are a process involving doctor and patient. The quality of case-taking and drug diagnosis therefore depends on the individual structure of both patient and doctor and on the given situation.

Summary

The quality of case-taking determines the reliability of the drug diagnosis. Distinguishing personal symptoms govern the search for the 'similar' drug. Before symptoms are evaluated, it is advisable to allow for a break, for a creative review to be gained through distance. In § 3 of the *Organon*, Hahnemann advises physicians to endeavour to get a clear image of the disease, of 'where healing is specifically needed'.

Perceiving the real illness means:
— knowing the 'idea inherent in a case of illness' (Eichelberger), the 'nature of the disorder' (Voisin)
— establishing the aetiology. Diagnosis of the illness.
— establishing an order based on current relevance and the given situation within the multi-layered disease process
— self knowledge as regards one's own strong and weak points, if necessary extending history-taking or using additional diagnostic measures.

2 Adaptation to the Given Situation

There is no one particular method to be used in all cases and by all homoeopathic physicians. Case-taking and drug diagnosis have to be individually adapted to the given situation. An acute cold or chronic migraine, a recent sprain or arthritis persisting for years — different jobs needs different tools. One thing which applies to all methods used to find the appropriate drug is that they must achieve their aim reliably and rapidly. In case of doubt the emphasis must be on 'reliably'.

It is important to aim for top quality in our work, yet another goal of equal importance is to give help to many individuals. We are not aiming for elistist medicine and would in fact starve to death in the present medical services system in Germany if we did not use methods that enable us to make quick decisions when choosing the appropriate drug, without, however, falling into the lazy habit of prescribing a mixture of drugs.

When the symptomatology is clear and obvious, the short route can be taken and will lead directly to our goal. It bases largely on getting a good synthetic overview and grasping the symptoms holistically; it requires a thorough knowledge of the drug pictures. Beginners may certainly use it where the symptomatology is clear and in the organotropic sphere. In cases lacking in clarity, with many strata, it will be necessary to analyse and evaluate the symptoms, usually with the aid of reference works (repertory and comprehensive materia medica). Kent in particular has developed the analytical method (repertorization) into a fine art. It is time-consuming and should be reserved for difficult cases, being the 'long route' to finding the appropriate drug. It will often prove effective where shorter routes prove inadequate for the purpose. Both routes should be known and used in accord with our ability and type of practice.

— **Learn the short routes, to give you time for the occasions when the long route has to be taken.**
— **Make your choice between the two possible methods entirely on the basis of the given situation and your own abilities.**
— **Do not get into the habit of using only the short route, perhaps from laziness.**

Always remember that homoeopathy is taylor-made and not off the peg. But a button can always be sown on again quickly.

3 Short Routes to Drug Diagnosis

WELL ESTABLISHED INDICATION
In some cases the spontaneous report given by the patient will immediately make it obvious that the shortest route can safely be taken. In this case the prescription is based on a well established indication (see p. 47).

Example
A pregnant woman reports that now, in her third month, her gums are bleeding. Otherwise she is well. Examination and blood status confirm her statement.
    Clinical diagnosis: *gingivitis gravidarum*.
    It is known from earlier consultations that there are no marked constitutional traits.
    Current prescription: *Mercurius solubilis* 12x bd.

This is a rapid and reliable route.[1]
    The reliability bases on the extensive experience generations of physicians have gained since 1800. Yet there is always need to be watchful and not to fall into complete routine. Problems are bound to arise if *Mercurius* is described in every case of bleeding gums.

CLINICAL PICTURE
This is given prime emphasis in textbooks on clinical homoeopathy and in training courses for homoeopathic physicians and for students. The route to drug diagnosis via the diagnosed disease makes homoeopathy more accessible; it relates to the organotropic and functiotropic actions of a number of homoeopathic drugs. Physicians totally geared to the familiar diagnosis who have not yet been able

to accept a phenomenological approach will find this route quite comprehensible. It makes it possible for anyone new to homoeopathy and also in daily practice to come to a rapid decision: a few characteristics (modalities, concomitants) make it possible to differentiate the appropriate drug among a limited number. It is legitimate to start from the clinical diagnosis on the road to drug diagnosis in situations where case-taking yields only few personal symptoms and the symptomatology is largely governed by the clinical condition. Acute infections come under this heading, as do the common cold, inflammatory conditions affecting the skin and mucosa taking their characteristic course. Hahnemann himself used relatively little individualization during the typhoid, cholera and scarlet fever epidemics which were part of his everyday experience in the field. He would then treat entirely on the basis of the *genius epidemicus*. If there is an influenza epidemic, for instance, we are able to treat the majority of patients effectively with just a handful of drugs such as *Aconitum, Belladonna, Gelsemium, Ferrum phosphoricum, Eupatorium* and *Bryonia*, saving ourselves and our patients a great deal of time.

It must be clearly stated, however, that we treat the patient, not the disease. The nature of the disease provides a conceptual framework for the nature of the presenting condition. We are in this case able to choose from a limited number of drugs which have proved their value on the basis of their toxicology, their tissue affinity, or their functional relationship in certain types of disease. Case-taking must however yield personal characteristics and modes of reaction, so that the one drug which is appropriate may be selected from the group. Personal symptoms lead to the choice of the particular drug. If someone were to ask us: 'Which drug do homoeopaths give in bronchitis?', we would have to ask them: 'Do you mean Mr Mayor's bronchitis or Mrs Smith's?' We all have our own way of coughing. Individual differences are always so considerable that any good practitioner, of whatever school, should make them his guideline in deciding on treatment. Sad to say, homoeopathy is more or less the only discipline where the patient's individual reaction is made the guideline.

Example
Main complaint: cough for 2 days.

O/E mucopurulent discharge running down back of throat, lungs clear. Diagnosis: retronasal catarrh.

Spontaneous report and specific questions: cough arises from irritation in throat, in constant brief bouts. Worse at night, better in a warm room, worse out of doors. Cold air discomforts. Covers mouth with scarf when outside. Fresh air feels very cold to him or her (outside temperature about 14°C).

Indirect questions: nothing further.

Drug diagnosis: starting from the clinical diagnosis of retronasal catarrh and taking into account the personal symptoms 'worse from cold air, inhaled air feels chilly' one arrives at *Corallium rubrum* 6x t.d.s.

Aids to drug diagnosis: textbooks of clinical homoeopathy (Stauffer, Voisin, Dorcsi's *Stufenplan*, Koehler's *Husten-Scriptum*).

AETIOLOGY

In the section on Aetiology in Chapter 4 reference was made to the importance of the triggering factor. The aetiology of an illness can quickly guide us to a group of drugs or even a particular drug if it emerges really clearly on case-taking. One thing everybody seems agreed on is that a clearly established aetiology makes drug diagnosis certain. Anyone wishing to arrive quickly at a good prescription should pay considerable attention to aetiological symptoms. The orthodox school often fiddles around with the 'causes' of diseases, always looking for new and 'even more causative causes',[2] and it keeps producing new drugs in its constant pursuit of the cause. From a philosophical point of view, our concept of aetiology is a purer one. We do not presume to uncover original causes.

An often heard criticism is that homoeopathy is symptomatic and not causal therapy. This merely shows the critic's ignorance of both homoeopathy and philosophy. The prime cause is outside the range of human perception. For those with religious beliefs, god is the prime cause of all subsequent 'causes'. In medicine, therefore, our range of perception does not go beyond the processes which ultimately triggered the illness, the *causa occasionalis* or *causa proxima*.

In the evolution of science, every age starts at a different point in determining the onset of a pathogenetic process, depending on the current state of knowledge. The fact that special significance attaches to aetiology in homoeopathic drug diagnosis makes it perfectly clear that we are just as interested in determining the immediate cause as the orthodox school. Where homoeopathic treatment is able to remove the susceptibility to infection it is 'more causal' than a form of treatment that applies only to the pathogen. If it is possible to cure loss of hair due to problems and worries with the appropriate 'worry' drug (*Acidum phosphoricum*) (see case history on p. 103), this takes more account of the cause than specific hair treatments which can only be symptomatic. I owe a great deal to Victor von Weizsaecker in this respect.

Knowledge of the triggering element in a process provides us with a guideline for taking action rather than theoretical discussion.

Example

Main complaint: headache, almost continuous.

Spontaneous report: from childhood recurrent headache in frontal region, very much worse last 4 years, since second concussion. First had been at age of 6; due to fall down stairs.

Indirect questions: headache with rush of blood to head and sensation of heat. Head very sensitive to exposure to sun.

Drug diagnosis: on the aetiology 'headache following concussion' four drugs with head trauma, *Arnica*, *Helleborus*, *Hypericum* and *Natrum sulphuricum*, rank highest for consideration.

Treatment: in this case *Arnica* 12x (8 drops b.d. for 3 weeks). Headaches better but not gone completely. *Arnica* 30x (once a week for 3 weeks) gave further improvement. Still a residue remaining. *Helleborus niger* LM VI (3 drops mane for 2 weeks, a week's break, then repeated).

Follow-up: no further headaches.

Books for consultation: Dorcsi *Stufenplan* II, Aetiology; textbooks of clinical homoeopathy (Stauffer, Koehler *Scriptum 'Physisches Trauma'*).

DRUG TYPES

Short routes to drug diagnosis in my view also include establishing the drug type on the basis of appearance.

It is a quick but risky route. It can be rewarding for physicians who train their eye and really look at their patients. There is, however, considerable risk of classifying people too rigidly. It is not the 'type' which is treated; the current illness is evaluated for its totality of symptoms and the prescription based on this. The totality of symptoms covers everything I hear from the patient and see when I look at him or her, i.e. the words spoken and the visible evidence of constitutional characteristics. Homoeopathy is a form of holistic medicine where particular attention is paid to the constitutional characteristics of patients.

The constitutional characterictics to be looked for are:

— Physique: round, bony, delicate, small, large, fat, thin
— Tissues: firm, flaccid, turgid, spongy
— Skin colour: pale, red, yellowy, greyish
— Hair colour: black, fair, brown, grey, red
— Skin temperature: warm, cold
— Skin type: dry, sweaty, coarse, large pores, delicate, transparent, smooth, wrinkled, clean, dirty
— Posture: upright, bent, tense, relaxed
— Gestures: controlled, expansive, trembling, calm, restless, tense, casual, slow, hasty
— Look: open, secretive, straight, oblique, cheerful, sad, composed, anxious.

It is possible to relate particular homoeopathic drugs to these visible characteristics of a person. Hahnemann in his day noted that some drugs acted particularly well if the patient was of a particular physical type.

Example
In his *Chronic Diseases* Part 4, under *Acidum nitricum*: 'This drug will be found to be of benefit more to patients of firm fibre (brunette) and less to those of flaccid fibre (blonde). It is also more suitable for chronic patients much tending to soft stools, being only rarely indicated in subjects who tend to be constipated.'

This observation, expanded and deepened by his successors, gave rise to the concept of drug types.

Beuchelt has presented these drug types very well, with excellent illustrations. Identity between a person and the drug he or she needs may be such that homoeopaths will speak of a *Calcarea carbonica* child, or of a *Sepia* type with reference to a woman. A domestic tyrant may be *Lycopodium* or a male *Nux vomica* type, with his jealous wife a *Lachesis*. The correspondence may be so close and so obvious that one may 'see' the drug which will cure by just considering the patient's appearance. But once again a warning must be given. If the current illness, often an acute disease, does not fit into the drug picture of the drug matching the type, only the currently indicated drug should be given. The type may be extremely well indicated, but before a prescription is made the case history must confirm any diagnosis based on appearance.

It is particularly in the field of paediatrics that drug types offer a good starting point in drug diagnosis, for here signs and attitudes are still presented without dissembling. Lymphatic children and their constitutional remedies *Calcarea carbonica*, *Calcarea phosphorica*, *Calcarea fluorica*, *Hepar sulphuris* and *Silicea* have many common and distinguishing characteristics and it is possible to choose the simile on the general impression of physique and behaviour plus the essence of the symptoms.

Example
A. Sch, a boy of 6.

Diagnosis based on appearance: plumpish boy, especially large abdomen, pale face, large head with bulging forehead, cold hands. Stands close to mother.

Main complaint: recurrent colds.

Spontaneous report: one cold follows another — tonsillitis, otitis twice, bronchitis. Stools only every third day; when he had a cold also diarrhoea with acid stools. Does not like school, wants to be with his mother all the time. Hardly ever plays with other children. Screams at night and then comes to mother, with his head sweaty on those occasions. Very sensitive skin. Facial eczema, worse from washing. Skin lesions fester for a long time.

O/E mucopurulent nasal discharge, tonsils enlarged, no inflammation. Cervical glands enlarged, soft. Bronchitic sounds at base. Skin feels cold, abdomen tympanitic, thick layer of abdominal fat, genitalia very small, wandering testicle. Teeth wide, second incisor small.

Specific questions: milk crust in infancy. In spite of vitamin D mild degree of rickets.

Indirect questions: milk intolerance, with diarrhoea after milk. Walked at 21 months. Late learning to speak. Several teeth carious.

Constitutional diagnosis: lymphatic type, with rickets, chilly, pale, hypogenital development.

Drug diagnosis: the habitus (short, broad, large head, bloated abdomen) and the constitutional signs of the lymphatic child (slow, chilly, pale) immediately point to the drug diagnosis of *Calcarea carbonica*. This is further borne out by a tendency to sweats on the back of the head, night terrors, clinging to mother, skin tending to eczema and festering, late walking and talking. Also inclination to be constipated and milk intolerance.

To recognize drug types in the physical make-up it is important to be thoroughly familiar with the constitutional drugs. In his *Children's Types*, Borland has given a very clear description of the way in which appearance and behaviour may be used as a basis for drug diagnosis in paediatric practice. Adults show typological characteristics less clearly, having been subject to a multiplicity of environmental factors over a long period of time — age, illnesses, traumas, conditions of life, occupation, stresses, fate.

KEY SYMPTOMS

Example

A new patient stated that she had been suffering from gastric pain for 20 years, with recurrent ulcers in the pyloric region and duodenum. Having heard this I decided to make another appointment for her to allow more time for case-taking in view of the length of her illness and many different treatments already received. Having got up from her chair her attention was caught by the view from the window where a huge crane was rotating as work was in progress on an underground garage behind the house. She took a step toward the window, looked down into the unexpectedly deep hole in the ground, and stepped back very quickly, saying: 'Oh, that is dreadful. It really pulls me to it.' This obvious phobic fear on looking down (high-rise syndrome) gave rise to a rapid question and answer sequence. 'Who cleans the windows of your flat?' 'My husband used to, now my daughter does it. I can't do such things.' 'Which floor are you on?' 'The second.' (That is the description used in Baden. In northern Germany and Great Britain it would be the first floor.) 'Would you like to move to a tower block where you'll have a beautiful view?' 'Heavens no, if I could really choose I'd live in a bungalow.' 'How about eructations?' 'A lot, but it all tenses up and won't come out properly. Sometimes I am almost exploding, it expands and grows big.'

Having obtained this confirmation, anyone familiar with the drug picture of *Argentum nitricum* would be able to be almost prophetic in describing her other symptoms to the lady.

Once one has experienced a key symptom in the patient, one never fails to be impressed by the sheer logical truth of homoeopathy. All niggling doubts and challenges offered by the scientific way of thinking are silenced when one has this experience. The successes achieved in this way and the almost instant attainment of a drug diagnosis give satisfaction to both patient and physician.

Not every key symptom is so well defined, however, that it acts like an open sesame and all is revealed. Clear and complete key symptoms are like the finger print of the perpetrator. The criminal police will of course have to go through their files to see if this particular print has been registered. We have to look through the repertory if the symptom is not known to us. It means that the short route via the key symptoms may turn out to be a long route, which may be embarrassing. Thorough study of principal signs and symptoms can save a great deal of time and sharpen the ear. We often only hear the things we are already familiar with out of the confusion of words making up the spontaneous report.

INTUITION

To conclude our discussion of short routes to drug diagnosis let us briefly consider the intuitive grasp of a patient and the drug he or she needs.

Many of the renowned figures in our profession are said to have an excellent 'clinical eye'. In the field of homoeopathy, too, one hears of physicians who had clear intuition and a real gift for discerning the appropriate drug after exchanging just a few words with the patient, and indeed often by just looking at him or her. Behind this intuition — and I do not deny it exists — one will, however, always find the immense amount of hard work put in by those highly gifted people. It is better to emulate such 'luminaries' by hard work, keeping a firm rein on our less brilliant intuitive gifts. Genuine facts — clear, rationally understandable symptoms presented by the patient — often provide a better basis for drug diagnosis. All 'maybe' and 'perhaps' is sloppy work. Proper aim must be taken if the target is to be hit. Julius Caesar is reported to have said *veni, vidi, vici* — I came, I saw, I conquered. Yet

Brutus struck him down after all. Perhaps we should reflect on this whenever we feel very sure of ourselves.

4 'Long Routes' to Drug Diagnosis

The decision as to whether a short or a long route will have to be taken in the individual case usually makes itself at the very beginning with anyone who has developed a good case-taking technique. If we follow the guidelines laid down by Hahnemann (*Organon* §§ 83-104) it will be obvious from the volume and quality of the spontaneous report given by the patient which route has to be taken. Those new to homoeopathy are advised at this point to go back and re-read the chapter on case-taking.

I think we all have to admit that laziness, pressure of time or a false sense of security often tempt us to try the short route first. We are in good company in this respect, for many judges are known to base their judgement on appearances. The result may be that the case has to be retried. We, too, have to go to the 'court of appeal' when we have made the wrong judgement — i.e. if the expected result has not been achieved. Taking the case again, and more thoroughly, we establish once again how the illness evolved. We must always look for the fault in ourselves when something goes wrong. The natural inclination is of course to blame others: it is the patient's fault; homoeopathy is no good; we ourselves are infallible of course.

The processing of material obtained through good quality case-taking presents a problem which has been the subject of considerable debate ever since Hahnemann's day. Every school of homoeopathy has its favourite method. V. Boenninghausen, Kent, Allen, Voisin (France), Dorcsi (Vienna), Eichelberger (Munich), Ortega, Paschero (South America) — the list of names illustrates the variety of methods.

Different methods have been developed because human nature varies — patients as well as doctors. Individual cases are many and varied — physicians are many and varied. Different materials call for different tools. Once we are aware of this it is obvious that no school can claim to have the only valid method. Any one method may be the right one in a particular case. What is important is that it gives reliable and rapid results. I am not in favour of generalization or of onesidedness. Keep an open mind, learn to use a number of different methods.

> We should never limit ourselves to a single school or the statements made by a single author. On the contrary, it is important to look everywhere for statements that seem serious and sensible and hold on to these if they are confirmed in practice . . . We must leave behind all rigid formulas; they are attractive in their simplicity but constantly contradicted by the rich variety of life and of illness. (Voisin [1960] p. 9 of German edition).

Cases show such wide variation and physicians have such a wide range of different gifts that the field of potential action opens out wide in all directions. There is plenty of scope for both the synthetic and the analytical approach. Intuition, art and solid craftsmanship have their potential and their limits. It is one of the joys of homoeopathy that its 'fullness' (to use Dorcsi's term) and depth are so great; there is room for apprentices, journeymen and masters and all can do good work. Differences between clinical homoeopathy, pure symptomatology, analytical repertorization, interpretation of 'mind' symptoms on the basis of depth psychology (Ortega, Paschero), a synthetic constitutional approach (Dorcsi) are irrelevant. Every route is equally valid. The route which in the individual case leads to rapid and sure success, i.e. to finding the simile, depends entirely on the quality of the material obtained on case-taking and also on the inclinations and nature of the physician, and his or her knowledge of materia medica. Our efforts to become masters are most likely to be successful if we follow the guidelines given in the *Organon*:

— **Individualization of every single case of illness (§ 83)**
— **Determining the totality of symptoms (§ 7)**
— **Selecting the really important symptoms according to the criteria given in § 153.**

This provides a secure basis for drug diagnosis. These basic requirements for any form of homoeopathic practice have never been in dispute. The differences between schools relate mainly to the way in which these requirements may be met.

It has been my experience in working with people new to homoeopathy, both doctors and students, and also from talking with 'old hands', that it is most important to consider these problems in more detail.

Many doctors and students have taught themselves, reading homoeopathic literature of different periods, written by different authors, representing different schools. The rich variety of views and suggestions will often make them unsure. Variety indicates the rich potential of a method. If, however, we develop differences of opinion on this basis we merely show ourselves to be narrow-minded and bigoted. When there are different interpretations it is often a good idea to go back to the source. Source studies yield more valuable information than secondary literature. That is a well-established fact.

Do read the original works of Hahnemann, even if the old-fashioned type of writing makes it difficult to start with. I regret to say I rather suspect that many of those who have produced the secondary literature have not fully taken in the original works, or they mix in a great deal of their own, making no clear distinction between their own ideas and those of others. This applies even to Kent.

Hahnemann is no sacred monument where we are concerned. But it is exactly because we are not simple 'believers' but assess our work critically for its results that we must not overlook the sources. Reading one of his many works one gets the feeling that he rather overestimated us, his successors, regarding our ability to understand. This overestimation has given rise to many differences among his followers. Hahnemann found it impossible to understand why his contemporaries did not spontaneously grasp and take up his ideas. He could not see that the instructions given in his *Organon of Practical Medicine* might not be adequate to base homoeopathic practice on. He should have described the method in such a way that we of the 'infant class' could have picked it up the way we learn how to write. Or, to use another image, Hahnemann set up the lighthouses marking the harbour entrance for those sailing the homoeopathic seas, but the charts we need to avoid running aground are inadequate. We see the goal but not always the way of reaching it safely. The goal is to find the simile. We do have the instructions given in §§ 7, 83 and 153 of the *Organon* to help us find the safe channel. Even in Hahnemann's own day, this was not enough for his students. In an 'Introductory Memorandum' to the second volume of his *Materia Medica Pura*, the master showed some degree of displeasure in the way he addressed his apprentices:

> Many people I know who have come half way on the road to homoeopathic medical practice have applied to me from time to time to make public more detailed comments as to how my teaching could be put to effect and how it should be applied in practice. It surprises me that after the clear instructions given in the *Organon of Practical Medicine* people can still ask for more specific directions.
>
> Another question I am asked is: 'How does one investigate the illness in every individual case?' As if the book in question did not contain sufficiently detailed information.[3]
>
> The inner process of therapy always bases on the principles which have already been stated. It cannot be made concrete and firmly established in every individual case, cannot be made more explicit by the story of a single cure, than has already been done in presenting the principles. Every case of non-miasmatic illness is peculiar and unique. And it is the uniqueness of it, that which distinguishes it from every other case, that belongs to it alone.[4]

Unfortunately this 'Introductory Memorandum' is not widely known, and this is one of the reasons why I am quoting it at some length. The other reason is a simple one: all secondary literature on drug diagnosis can be assessed to see if it really is a great deal better and offers real advantages. Those claiming to be followers of Hahnemann and then taking their own road after all, must allow us to ask them why they choose to do so. If they have good and fair reason and achieve convincing results we will of course accept this. It is not a question of being purists, idolators or of clinging rigidly to established traditions. It is not a question of Hahnemann as a person, but entirely of 'rapidly, gently and lastingly' restoring to health the patients entrusted to our care. (*Organon* § 2)

Every reliable method of drug diagnosis must take its orientation from the three basic requirements referred to above. They are so important that we have good reason to repeat them:
— Individualization of every single case of illness
— Determining the totality of symptoms
— Selecting the really important symptoms according to the criteria given in § 153 of the *Organon*.

INDIVIDUALIZATION

In deciding on the short or the long route to drug diagnosis we are adapting to the given situation. The decision is made on an objective basis. Personal, subjective elements (laziness, pressure of time, lack of sympathy) are as far as possible eliminated. The personal gifts utilized in the evaluation of the symptomatology are part of the individual freedom a physician brings to the cognitive process. Homoeopathic drug diagnosis ranges from good craftsmanship to artistic intuition.

In straightforward cases, the cognitive process may be limited to a cross-section of the current problem. It will need to go further than this, however, whenever the individual situation of the patient calls for the longitudinal section of medical biography.

TOTALITY AND SUM AND ESSENCE OF SYMPTOMS

The history ranges widely in order to get as comprehensive a view as possible of the totality of symptoms. This has already been discussed in the chapter on Symptomatology. For present purposes, that thread will be taken up again and an attempt made to penetrate to a deeper level.

Example
A patient presented with pain in the shoulder and back.

Spontaneous report: frequent lancinating pain in shoulder and back, sometimes as if from a knife.

Specific questions: pains had persisted for about 18 months, worse on moving the right arm and taking a deep breath. No obvious aetiology. Factor at work? His work involved sitting at an assembly line and making monotonous movements with the right arm.

Examination: arms and neck freely mobile, myogelosis in paravertebral region between C4 and Th7, more marked on right, increased sensitivity to pressure in region of right shoulder blade, max. in point at margin of scapula close to lower angle. Lung n.a.d.

Comment: these local signs and symptoms were not enough to establish the drug diagnosis. The totality of symptoms had to be determined. Treatment where one has the whole person in one's sights is more demanding. The short route could not be taken in this case. The phenomena noted so far did not make it possible to perceive the illness. What was the significance of the pain in the shoulder? Was it enough to label this a shoulder-arm syndrome? In this case it was necessary to continue with:

Indirect questions: (head-to-foot system): frequent eye inflammations with lacrimation, redness of conjunctiva, his eye specialist had prescribed drops for him but these only helped for a time. Head felt dull, with pressing frontal pain, especially above the right eye. When tired roaring noise in ear; generally tired easily, fell asleep sitting in his chair at night; woke quite often between 3 and 4 a.m. with pain in right epigastrium, 'as if something were contracting there'. Better on getting up and eating a little, went and got himself a piece of bread. Pain radiating to back and right shoulder. In the mornings, rheumatic pain in thigh, felt stiff. Feet cold, especially the right foot.

Stools: occasional diarrhoea after rich foods, more commonly constipation with nodular stools, ineffectual urging. Clayey stools.

Desires and dislikes relating to food: liked warm milk which relieved stomach symptoms. Rich foods produced fullness and pressure in epigastrium.

Frame of mind: often depressed and irritable, would get annoyed at trifles and get into a rage.

Evaluation: The totality of symptoms presented a rich picture in this case. This fullness of symptoms does not emerge if a case is considered within the limited confines of a specialist discipline. An orthopaedic specialist would only get part of the picture, a gastroenterologist another part of the same picture. The eye specialist would only be concerned with the conjunctivitis, the ear specialist with the roaring in the ear. Each treats the patient from his standpoint, and the diagnosis will be in terms of his specialist field. A homoeopathic physician takes a holistic approach and the need for a drug diagnosis relating to the whole person directs his attention to the totality of signs and symptoms. In the case described above, the 'diagnosis' would be *Chelidonium majus*. It is not what we would normally call a 'diagnosis' in terms of pathological anatomy, but takes into account the totality of functional disorder in the case before him. We know that *Chelidonium* has the liver and gall bladder as the principal point of attack. The epigastric symptoms with pain radiating to the right shoulder blade and right supraorbital region and the cold right foot are part and parcel of this, as is the 'bile' shown in the patient's emotional reactions.

Hahnemann spoke of the 'totality of symptoms' and also of the 'sum and essence' of symptoms (*Organon* § 18).

'Totality' refers more to the completeness of the symptomatology, whilst 'sum and essence' relates to the quality of what comes to expression. In other words, we need to have a large volume of material if we are to find the elements that are of real value. Leers put it in very descriptive terms: 'We need to shovel a great deal of sand in order to find the grains of gold.' Nash referred to the totality of symptoms as the *tout ensemble*:

> In actual practice there are two kinds of cases that come to every physician. One is the case that may be prescribed for with great certainty of success on the symptoms that are styled *characteristic* and *peculiar* (*Organon* § 153). The other is where in all the case there are no such symptoms appearing; then there is only one way, viz., to hunt for the remedy that, in its pathogenesis, contains what is called the '*tout ensemble*' of the case. The majority of cases, however, do have standing out like beacon lights, some characteristic or keynote symptoms which guide to the study of the remedy that has the whole case in its pathogenesis. [5]

In theory it would be possible to use the totality of symptoms unselected by making the drug diagnosis with the aid of a suitably programmed computer. Poorly differentiated symptoms mean a wide range of possible drugs. Poor differentiation means little potential for making distinction. The rubric in the repertory will be correspondingly large. Large rubrics require so much time to copy out that technical aids are essential. A punched card system may be used as a kind of mini-computer (Boger, Leers). Details of the method will be discussed in the next chapter. At this point is suffices to say that using large rubrics one almost always arrives at major drugs, i.e. polychrests (*Sulphur, Arsenicum, Lycopodium* a.o.). Statistical probability suggests that drugs with many well-known symptoms will come up most frequently in the large rubrics. Less well-known drugs with few but highly characteristic symptoms go through the net. This is the reason why it is essential to make a selection from the totality of symptoms. The resulting concentrate of essential symptoms is the 'sum and essence' of symptoms. It includes all statements and signs characteristic of the patient and his individual illness.

SELECTION AND EVALUATION OF SYMPTOMS

The totality of symptoms provides the raw material for drug diagnosis. A selection is made to arrive at the sum and essence of symptoms. The patient's spontaneous report with its free flow of associations often presents a confusion of diagnostic terms he or she has read about, commonplaces, and valuable personal statements. Signs and symptoms are only of value if accurately defined. The ideal are complete symptoms. They provide the basis on which similarity between disease picture and drug picture can be established. All this is perfectly clear; the real problem lies in the detail. This we have to find a way of dealing with. Our method of working may be compared to the search for incriminating evidence, often a problem to the criminal police. The criminal is only rarely caught in the act. The traces he leaves, the circumstances involved, the tools — all these may be of value. Criminal investigation covers everything from the ideal (the actual perpetrator) to the minimum, the faintest trace which may be evidence.

When we try to find the appropriate drug in everyday homoeopathic practice we are also in a situation somewhere between the ideal and the minimum possible. In some cases the patient's situation, his or her signs and symptoms are so obvious, clear and complete that the experienced physician feels real satisfaction in perceiving the similarity to a drug picture and noting the rapid results. In another case one finds oneself in constant danger of getting stuck. A little bit of a sign here, a fragment there, contradictory modalities, unclear aetiology, clinically n.a.d., biography yielding nothing. The process of making the drug diagnosis lies between those two poles of fullness and consistency on the one hand and symptoms both scarce and indefinite on the other.

THE ESSENTIALS OF A CASE

The first question to be asked concerns the essentials (see p. 87). Before we make our choice based on the ranking value of symptoms we must look for the thread running through the whole case history. We need to grasp the 'idea inherent in a case of illness' (Eichelberger).

Examples
O.S., a woman of 32. Main complaint: loss of hair.

Spontaneous report: had been treated by skin specialist for a long time, was even given a homoeopathic drug which she proudly presented: *Thallium* 6x. No result.

Specific questions: loss of hair for 6 months, hair lost by the handful, tired easily. Nothing of real value in this. Indirect questioning finally brought us to the 'idea' in the case: She had had problems and worries concerning her mother for the last 6 months.

The aetiology 'due to problems and worries' suggested *Acidum phosphoricum*. This gave an immediate improvement over the next 6 weeks and also cured her tiredness.

Comment: the aetiology of a disorder will often take us to essentials.

A. Schl., a man of 60, medium size, well-built, broad-shouldered. Main complaint: cough with difficulty in breathing.

Spontaneous report: very short of breath, worse walking, particularly uphill or up stairs; better when at rest, coughs in a warm room.

Specific questions: expectoration for last 6 months, yellowy grey. Cough better in open air.

Indirect questions: sweats in bed, towards morning.

Examination: plenty of moist rales at base, percussion note hyper-resonant. Cor n.a.d., bp 160/90.

Diagnosis: emphysema/bronchitis.

Treatment: initially *Quebracho* 2x, without results, then *Calcarea carbonica* 12x.

At the third consultation, specific questions were put once again as to whether there had been anything special 6 months previously, when the bronchitis started. So far the answer had been negative, but now he remembered that he had been to see a dermatologist about a month before that, because of a skin rash. He had been given a lotion to apply externally and the irritation had soon subsided.

This suggested *Sulphur* 6x and 10 days later the cough and dyspnoea had greatly improved.

Comment: The essential point was a shift from the skin inwards following external applications. The search for a suppressant mechanism will often put us on the right track for the drug that will give a complete cure.

U. E., a woman of 36, pasty, light-brown hair. Main complaint: pain on micturition.

Spontaneous report: burning pain with frequent urging for a week, the burning sensation is described spontaneously and with emphasis.

Indirect questions: she had got her feet wet a week ago and felt very cold.

Examinations: just positive for protein, sugar negative, UBG normal, sediment leuco +++, mucus, nitrite negative, bacteria positive.

Treatment: following well-established indication for severe burning pain, *Cantharis* 6x 5 drops t.d.s.

Follow-up: rapid improvement. Urine: leuco +, bacteria negative.

Six weeks later the patient returned. Main complaint now: a cold.

Spontaneous report: had had a cold for 3 days, often had colds. Secretion watery at first, then purulent. No temperature. Anterior nares slightly red, much sneezing, better in the open.

Treatment: based on the clinical picture: *Allium cepa* 6x.

Two weeks later the patient returned again. Her cold was better, but it had dragged on over week — she was used to this. She now wanted to be referred to a gynaecologist as she had a discharge. Referral.

Report: polyp at the os, cyst in left ovary.

The gynaecologist had suggested surgery.

The patient came back to me to ask if an operation could not be avoided. Case taken again. Result: definitely sycotic constitution (see p. 201). The essential element in this case was the underlying constitutional weakness. The manifestations in different organs were merely 'tips of the iceberg', there was a consistent underlying diathesis. Treatment based on this: *Thuja* LM VI, followed by LM XIV and LM XVIII.

Comment: the drug diagnosis for individual morbid changes had been based on an apparent similarity that struck the eye. The example has been deliberately chosen. It is a confession of having done the wrong thing, missing the essential point by not considering constitution and diathesis.

The above examples served to indicate that essential symptoms can only be found with a good case-taking technique. They also show that history-taking is a process starting from the patient's main complaint and continuing on to the 'heart' of the disorder. It sometimes takes considerable patience to follow this course. Spontaneously mentioned phenomena are always of value. Squeezing the patient dry not only shows lack of tact but also tends to lead into blind alleys. It is sometimes better to resolve a case step by step rather than try and achieve optimum results in a first rush.

The examples also show that the question as to the essential point in a case of illness determines the selection of symptoms. Essential and accurately defined symptoms are the sum and essence of symptoms. Selection immediately eliminates symptoms which tell us nothing about the person or the nature of the morbid disorders. Statements of no value are those made in very general terms or merely hinted at (e.g. tiredness, listlessness, loss of appetite) or diagnostic labels such as vegetative dystonia, circulatory disorder. Value attaches only to information that aids drug diagnosis by providing differentiation. The more precise a statement the better. It should be remembered that complete symptoms are the ideal. The precision of a statement is also determined by the way it is uttered. All symptoms mentioned spontaneously and with emphasis, all symptoms persisting for a long time and continuing to get worse require greater attention. Symptoms mentioned in response to questions on the other hand, and older symptoms which have rather tended to get better to date, are of less importance, unless they relate to constitution and diathesis. All statements made by a patient using the same or similar terms for different organic regions are of value.

In the chapter on Symptomatology it was said that all symptoms and signs ranking more as general symptoms, i.e. involving the whole person, carry more weight than local symptoms. Let me repeat what was said in that chapter (p. 38):

> The totality of symptoms is obtained by history-taking, observation and examination. A certain order will emerge on evaluation of the total

material. This order is based on the hierarchic order of the person: phenomena relating to soul and spirit come before those relating to the body; anything relating to the whole person comes before local symptoms; anything specific to the individual is rated higher than anything one would normally expect to see with a particular disease.

That is the general rule which has proved its value over and over again. We should not make it an absolute or a matter of routine, however. Phenomena relating to soul and spirit do rank highest, but it is only possible to evaluate and structure data one has actually obtained on history-taking. Two common errors have to be considered here. Firstly, putting too high a value on symptoms relating to mind and intellect, and secondly forgetting that there are no negative symptoms.

Example
In the presence of a medical student who had already taken the second course in homoeopathy, I prescribed *Graphites* in a case of eczema. He asked me why I had prescribed *Graphites*, for the patient was neither lazy, nor chilly, fat or a greedy eater, nor did he seem inert. I agreed that the patient had not shown these characteristics, yet the morphological appearance of the skin had shown exact correspondence to *Graphites*: Fissures and desquamation, also burning sensations in the skin, worse from heat, particularly warmth of bed; localization in the flexures of the elbows, behind the ears and around the lid margins had also been characteristic. All the positive signs of *Graphites* action had been present. It was true, the wider consititional similarity had not been there, nor the mental symptoms of the drug. This needed to be taken into account in choosing the potency. The 7c gave rapid improvement. If there had been full agreement also with regard to constitution and indicative mental symptoms it would have been possible to prescribe the 30c or an LM potency.

Significance does not attach to anything missing from the total picture. The drug diagnosis must logically be based on the signs and symptoms which are present. This applies to all spheres, including the mentals. In almost every case we find only part of the drug picture. The high ranking order of mental and intellectual symptoms particularly comes into its own when a final decision has to be made between two or three drugs.

Example
In a chronic case I was undecided between *Arsenicum* and *Phosphorus*. These two drugs can be very similar in symptoms and behaviour. Gentle discussion on the subject of thoughts of suicide got the patient to say that she had made an 'attempt' 3 years earlier, with sleeping pills, as she felt one night that there was no way out from the situation she was in. She had first intended to open her veins, but sleeping pills seemed 'better' from an aesthetic point of view.

This made it easy to decide for *Arsenicum* and against *Phosphorus*, because of 'suicide with poison or knife'.

If really convincing mental symptoms place a drug among those for final consideration it is generally admissible to overlook lack of total agreement in local symptoms. Local changes are the product of a central disruption in vital powers.

Summary

Good case-taking will often yield a number of signs and symptoms from which to choose. Precise statements are always important for the drug diagnosis. Symptoms referred to spontaneously and with certainty rank high, especially if they have been worse recently. Older symptoms continue to have significance in the context of biography and constitution if the current disorder shows a definite link with the constitutional terrain. The ranking value of symptoms is based on the hierarchy of the person: parts are maintained whithin the whole and controlled from the sphere of soul and spirit. Personal aspects stand out above those that are collective.

Drug diagnosis bases mainly on phenomena expressing the individual reactions of the patient. This is in accord with § 153 of the *Organon*. In a special case it is also possible for local symptoms to be *unusual*. In another case, individual character lies in *peculiar* mental symptoms. A third case may have *remarkable* general symptoms. It goes against the essential requirement of treating each case as individual to make the hierarchy of symptoms a routine matter.

The precision of symptoms and their ranking value in the hierarchy of the person together determine their value for drug diagnosis. Some authors treat the hierarchy of symptoms too rigidly. The danger inherent in this is that drugs are ignored which have very precise individual symptoms but not sufficiently well-known general symptoms ranking high in the hierarchy of the person. These 'lesser drugs' do not get proper attention if we concentrate exclusively on the numerous general symptoms of the polychrests (widely used drugs with a wide range of action such as *Sulphur*).

Example
A patient with multiple sclerosis who had achieved a long period of remission with *Phosphorus*, was about to go into an acute stage again. She reported hypersensitivity to the least noise; sensation in the thigh as if something were contracting and then letting go again, especially if the leg got cold. Kent lists (*Asarum Europaeum* under 'Sensitive, noise, to' (p. 79), Contraction/Cramps, thigh' (pp. 967 and 974), 'Spasmodic' (p. 974). The drug picture confirmed this and the drug was prescribed in the 6x. Ten days later the patient reported marked improvement. She stayed in remission.

It is evident from this example that the quality of symptoms has to be assessed from two angles, i.e. their precision and their ranking value in the hierarchy of the person. A high rank in the hierarchy and top quality and precision are the height of prefection. Chess players will know that a pawn can play a vital role if in the right position.

A drug must not be excluded from consideration because characteristic mental or general symptoms are absent or cannot be elicited in a particular case. *There are no negative symptoms.* The quality of a symptom depends on its precision and its rank in the hierarchy of the person.

Table 3: Criteria on Which Selection is Based in Making the Drug Diagnosis

Precision of Symptoms
1   Characteristic, striking and unusual symptoms
2   Symptoms mentioned spontaneously and with emphasis
3   Complete symptoms
4   Symptoms persisting for a long time and getting worse — particularly if orientated towards constitution and diathesis
5   New symptoms which are getting worse.

Ranking Order
1   Aetiology
2   Mental and intellectual symptoms
3   General symptoms relating to the whole person
   a) Sensations and modalities involving the whole person
   b) Sexuality, menses
   c) Cravings, desires and dislikes relating to foods
   d) Nature of excretions and secretions
   e) Sleep and dreams
4   Symptoms relating to individual organs, local symptoms with modalities and concomitant symptoms.

5 Problems with Drug Diagnosis

Drug diagnosis may present problems if there are two few symptoms or too many.

FEW SUBJECTIVE SYMPTOMS

Particular patience is required with patients who produce hardly any reasonable personal symptoms or in cases where a verbal statement cannot be obtained: unconscious patients, the mentally ill, infants,[6] people too lazy to talk who hold the optimistic view that the doctor knows it all anyway, organic disease if decompensated.

If there is organic disease, the symptoms mainly relate to the pathological changes and consequent loss of function. Most of these patients have already had a variety of treatments, often heroic, and it is difficult to distinguish between the side effects of drugs, the consequences of suppression, and organic lesions. *Nux vomica* (drug-induced problems) or *Sulphur* (suppression of eliminatory processes) may on occasion help to clarify the situation. It is sometimes still possible to help patients who have been on immunosuppressive therapy for long periods or suffer the consequences of suppressed pyrexia. (Kent's 'Reaction, lack of' and 'Quinine, abuse of', both on p. 1397, correspond to todays suppression of fever, sequelae of immunosuppression.) The well-established organotropic drugs also come into their own here, given in low potency. It will be possible at least to achieve palliation; genuine cures are rare.

We should always keep heart, however, never abandoning patients to their fate and giving up all hope. On the other hand we must not cloud the issue with lies. Truth coupled with hope will give strength. One person will need to be given more hope, of course, another more truth. Again the principle which applies in homoeopathy proves important: individualize, never use a routine approach.

People too lazy to talk are made to utter by getting them to fill in a questionnaire. 'Indisposed to talk, desire to be silent, taciturn' may in itself be a symptom (Kent p. 86). 'Reluctant to reply' may be found in Dorcsi's *Symptomenverzeichnis*, p. 91.

Objective signs have particular significance where verbal statements cannot be obtained (unconscious patients etc.). This is where the trained eye comes into its own, and the ability to take a synthetic approach. All one's sense organs need to be alive — see, smell, touch, sense to obtain objective signs and compare these with the toxicological data of drug action.

Example
A boy of 17 collapsed after a 100-metre run at a sporting event. He was lying on the ground, whey-faced, pulse small, hard and thready, pinched face, retching, cold sweat, eyes closed. People wanted to cover him, but he pushed the blanket away. This is a situation where only the signs speak: collapse, pale face, cold sweat, nausea, retching, eyes closed, hard, thready pulse, does not want to be covered.

Veratrum album and *Tabacum* are the two drugs to be considered for collapse. The hard, thready pulse, aversion to being covered, nausea and desire to keep eyes closed pointed to *Tabacum*. *Veratrum* has a weak pulse, wants warmth, has more cold sweat on forehead.

After a dose of *Tabacum* 30c the young athlete soon felt better. A fellow club member said to him: 'There you have it! I told you to keep off those cigarettes.' Such corroboration from someone 'not in the know' is excellent confirmation that the right drug was chosen. The aetiology of this collapse, and I could not possibly have known this, was nicotine consumption prior to physical exertion.

In the case of infants and small children the drug diagnosis is often based on objective signs in conjunction with the symptomatology obtained from a reference person (father, mother). Drug typology and constitutional characteristics can sometimes make us independent of any form of verbal statement.

MANY SIGNS AND SYMPTOMS

Talkative patients. Sometimes one wants to throw up one's hands in horror during the spontaneous report, for the floodgates are opened. It is all bubbling up, the fountain leaps to and fro, and everything gives, like a jellyfish. If you try to get it down on paper — it's been and gone already, the flow goes on. Selection of symptoms? Which? If it proves impossible to bring some order into the symptoms, the striking symptom of loquacity may itself be used in drug diagnosis. The individual way of putting things, the personal variety of loquacity can point to the appropriate drug.[7]

VARIABLE SYMPTOMS

In some cases the spontaneous report may sound confusing because statements appear to be contradictory: sometimes like this, sometimes like that, now here, now there. If variability is almost the rule we may think of *Ignatia, Pulsatilla; Sulphur* with its wide-ranging symptomatology (psora) and *Psorinum* also tend to be confusing, as is *Tuberculinum*. The elimination of toxins via the skin, mucosa, intestine and kidneys produces variable symptoms.

Here Constitution and Diathesis are the principles on which order may be based. Constitutional weaknesses must be tracked down. The medical biography provides the pointers we need. The medical biography of the chronically sick will reveal characteristic morbid processes, and the many and varied symptoms will be ascribable to these. Establishing order on the basis of constitution and diathesis we achieve a basic structure. Direction is given to elements that appear to be going off in different directions. Constitution and diathesis will be discussed in more detail in a later chapter.

In cases of chronic and constantly recurring disease it is important to establish the constitutional background to the many varied pathological, functional and mental symptoms. Tinkering around with isolated pathological phenomena will not take us beyond the periphery, it is merely palliative or cosmetic. We will be fundamentally unable to achieve a cure.

6 Avoidable Errors

Hahnemann had a point when he said: 'Copy, but copy exactly.' It has been my definite experience, further confirmed by checking, by tests and in conversation with colleagues, that the best results and most reliable results are obtained if we follow the guidelines for drug diagnosis given in the *Organon*.

From my own mistakes (and we all make mistakes, over and over again) and through teaching activity I have tried to learn where the underwater cliffs and shallows lie, to know the common errors that can be avoided.

PRESCRIBING ON THE DIAGNOSIS

Homoeopathy is a phenomenological method. Drug diagnosis must take its orientation from observed phenomena (symptoms and signs). No other physician since Hippocrates has based his approach to treatment as clearly on the specific individual phenomena as Hahnemann has done. We must come away from thinking rigidly in terms of explaining the illness, the way we have been trained, and gain the freedom we need to observe the patient. The thinking processes used to work out an explanation are retrograde and analytical, going from B to A. The approach is unicausal, and it has its rightful place and its triumphs in the sphere of mechanical processes. Observation of the phenomena on the other hand encompasses the whole, encompasses multicausal processes in nature. Complex natural processes cannot be traced to single causes. Analytical thinking aims to resolve multiplicity into individual lines capable of explanation. In certain areas, e.g. infectious diseases, scientific medicine has achieved undoubted successes by reducing pathological processes to a single 'cause'. In many other areas it comes up against its limits and fails to understand that the problem lies in the wrong line of thinking.

This had to be said, for it is the background to the first of the avoidable errors which consists in ignoring the phenomena, becoming attached to the diagnosis as a collective, abstract concept. It is the reason why many homoeopathic colleagues give preference to organotropic drugs. It also is the only possible explanation why many who practise homoeopathy as well as conventional medicine cannot do without compound drugs. Compound prescriptions still have a nice 'umbilical cord' linking them to the diagnosis, to the collective approach, to the explanation of disease. A physician basing himself on the phenomenology will in every single case face the decision as to which individual drug corresponds to the symptoms of this one patient. He has decided in favour of observing the patient and of the individual patient as a person. He puts his trust in the guidance given by the totality of signs and symptoms.

Example
Typical phenomena of *Belladonna* are: red, hot, swollen, throbbing sensations.

These are the outstanding phenomena to be taken into account for drug diagnosis in the following pathological conditions which can be differentiated diagnostically:

Table 4

Name of disease (diagnosis)	Explanation of disease (cause)	Observation of patient (phenomena)
acute febrile infection	bacteria, viruses	face bright red, hot, sweating, wants to keep covers on, throbbing of carotids
sunstroke	hyperaemia of meninges	face bright red, hot, temporal arteries congested, throbbing; may be disorientated, confused, frightening hallucinations, pupils dilated
fresh boil	bacteria	bright red swelling in circumscribed area, throbbing pain
nappy rash	fungi, bacteria	skin bright red and shiny, taut, swollen

Moral: Stick to the phenomena.

ILLNESS NOT FULLY RECOGNIZED

Stick to the phenomena was our last 'battle cry'. Yes indeed, but not blindly so. Individual phenomena may deceive unless they are seen in the full context of the symptomatology. The totality of symptoms also covers all the circumstances which point to the genesis, the evolution of a disorder. A complete symptom must always include the aetiology. The totality of symptoms and the aetiology reveal the particular illness, and additional data are obtained on examination. Individual phenomena find their rightful place within this totality. Analytical thinkers are often in danger of pouncing on individual symptoms and wanting to track them down in reference works (repertories). Many a Kentian who has not fully understood Kent, his teacher, may be accused of this, making repertorization an aim in itself. An incomplete symptom (no aetiology) may lead to completely different treatments, failing to find the simile.

Table 5 provides an example. It is a synopsis based on a number of case histories.

Table 5

Symptom	Aetiology	Recognized illness	Possible therapy
Lancinating pain in nape and occiput, better resting and from warmth	1 Trauma of cerv. spine	Vertebrae blocked due to whiplash injury	Osteopathy, *Rhus tox.*
	2 Eyestrain	Accommodation problem	Glasses, *Onosmodium*, *Ruta*
	3 Nape getting chilled	Occipital neuralgia after washing hair	*Belladonna*
	4 Rheumatic? Wear?	Arthritis of spine	Massage, *Cimicifuga*, *Lachnanthes*

DRUG PROCESSES NOT FULLY KNOWN

We often fail to see the full significance of symptoms as regards their evolution. Illness is a process ranging from mild indisposition to the final burnt-out state (usually only few symptoms). Drug symptoms fit into a similar process, ranging from the subtle symptomalogy more determined by individual reactivity, to manifest organic lesions and finally the crude destruction evident in the toxicology. Illness and drug action are dynamic processes following a similar course. We take the case and initiate treatment at some point or other in a process which runs in time and may develop one way or another. The materia medica presents the whole picture of drug action from initial subtle effects to reactive sequelae and the final stage known to us from toxicology. It is not reasonable to expect the total drug picture to be available for comparison when making the drug diagnosis for an acute condition at the local stage. In a particular instance we will only find the part of the picture corresponding to the present, as yet limited, situation.

A drug must not be excluded because an apparently important element is missing in the case in question. There are no negative symptoms.

Examples
The choice of *Arnica* to treat a haematoma can be safely based on aetiology (contusion, crush injury), the appearance of the traumatized part (red, possibly blue or green), the sensation (as if battered) and the modalities (painful to touch, in damp cold). The wider spectrum of the *Arnica* picture will emerge only with infections like typhoid or in a case of apoplexy.

A number of further *Arnica* symptoms may be present in a case of apoplexy (cerebrovascular accident):

Head bright red; stupor, responds if spoken to but immediately relapses into indifference again; wants to be left alone, sending doctor and nurses away saying he needs no help; does not want to be touched; confused, vertigo on closing eyes; involuntary defecation during sleep; frightening dreams; keeps turning in bed, cannot find a comfortable position as bed seems too hard.

Alternatively we may remember only the initial stages of drug action, forgetting the final stage.

Example
Calcarea carbonica is almost exclusively used in the treatment of pasty, lymphatic small children. The drug does, however, offer a wide spectrum of signs in the ageing — sclerosis, hypertension, lithaemia, polyps, myomas.

We also tend to cling too much to the physical type of the rather plump *Calcarea carbonica* child, failing to consider the dystrophic child with Mach's syndrome where the only signs and symptoms indicative of *Calc. carb.* are the distended abdomen, the sensitivity to cold, sour sweats and diarrhoea, intolerance of milk and fear of being left alone.

PERSONAL PREFERENCES
Hahnemann's advice was that we must be faithful and unprejudiced, i.e. proof against temptation, when recording the patient's symptoms in case-taking. If we do so and yet keep coming up with the same familiar drugs, this serves to indicate that we are not individualizing sufficiently. Case-taking should not be 'angled' towards a favourite drug. We do not see what we do not want to see. Every 'searcher' finds what he or she is looking for.

RIGID ROUTINE IN ESTABLISHING RANKING ORDER
It is correct to say that 'mind' symptoms rate high in drug diagnosis. Yet this applies only in a fully developed morbid state and there are limitations if we are dealing with local syndromes of recent origin.

Antimonium crudum is very effective in the treatment of plantar warts. Yet this is a local syndrome involving only the skin and one therefore cannot expect to find the irritability, anger at every little attention and thick, milky-white coating on the tongue which are important principal symptoms in gastric disorders.

Every single case presents only part of the whole drug picture. It is important to make sure this part exactly matches the chosen drug.

PREMATURE DECISIONS

We all of us tend to be in too much of a hurry and stick at a single unusual or striking symptom. This one grain of gold is then dressed up to make it a key symptom, angling the whole of our case-taking in the desired direction. The desire to find a short route can easily turn into a compulsion to reach the goal quickly with the help of a well-established indication. We all tend to work too quickly on the basis of preconceived ideas: throat feels constricted — immediately the pen writes *Lachesis*; better from movement? — that is *Rhus tox.*; vertigo when looking to the side — *Conium* of course. I cannot see any difference between this kind of prescribing and the prescription of painkillers for headaches or the use of compound drugs on the principle 'Coughex' for a cough and 'Fluex' for influenza.

PREFERENCE GIVEN TO LOCAL SYMPTOMS

The history usually starts with a local symptom. This main symptom has to be fully taken in. Our search for the appropriate drug should not stop at this point, however. It is always necessary to establish the totality of symptoms, and it is only in rare cases that a single local symptom dominates the whole morbid process. We need to remember over and over again that the affected part of the organism is only part of the whole. 'All parts of the organism are intimately bound up with each other, forming an indivisible whole in our perceptions and functionally.' (*Organon* § 189) And 'Genuine treatment applied by a physician to a disorder which has arisen in external parts of the body should therefore be directed to the whole, to the annihilation and cure of the general malady . . . , if it is to be effective, reliable, thorough and helpful.' (*Organon* § 190)

It is evident therefore that we do not base treatment on a local process the way a specialist would. Drug diagnosis relying entirely on a local symptom is a mere 'symptomatic cover-up' and cannot achieve a lasting cure.

7 Summary

The reliability of a drug diagnosis depends on the quality of case-taking. Without a good history there can be no therapy.

A number of different routes are available for drug diagnosis and a choice has to be made on the basis that the chosen route will rapidly and safely lead to the goal. Different routes are determined by the extent of the disorder, and they may be long or short.

The individual physician with his knowledge of materia medica and individual gifts relating to the analytical or synthetic approach to symptomatology has a number of free choices in making his or her decisions.

A synthetic grasp is possible if symptoms are clear and many. Vague and fragmentary symptoms force us to use the analytical approach.

Before the physician evaluates the symptoms revealed by the patient an effort should be made to grasp the 'nature of the disorder'. Recognition of the nature of the illness makes the ordering and valuation of symptoms and signs meaningful.

Homoeopathic physicians are able to avoid error by following the dictum of Hahnemann: 'Copy, but copy exactly.' To copy exactly means to base the drug diagnosis on § 153 of the *Organon*:

> In choosing the homoeopathic drug specific to the case, particular and almost exclusive attention must be given to the more remarkable, peculiar, unusual and singular (characteristic) symptoms . . . ; symptoms closely similar to these in particular must be present among those of the drug we are looking for, if it is to be the one most appropriate for achieving a cure.

[1]   This reliable indication may be found in Hochstetter [1973], p. 105.
[2]   This formulation has been taken from a lecture given by A. Braun, Harlaching nr Munich.
[3]   Hahnemann, *Materia Medica Pura* vol. 2, p. 27.
[4]   Ibid., vol. 2, pp. 30-1.
[5]   Nash EB. *Leaders in Homoeopathic Therapeutics*, 4th edn. p. 22. Philadelphia: Boericke & Tafel 1913.
[6]   For particular aspects of paediatrics, see Imhaeuser and Foubister.
[7]   See Kent p. 63; Dorcsi *Symptomenverzeichnis* p. 98. Special study on the subject: Gnaiger J.

7

DRUG DIAGNOSIS USING
A REPERTORY

The number of drug symptoms is vast and a repertory has to be used to obtain confirmation.

Von Boenninghausen and Kent evolved a special technique of choosing the appropriate drug by making analytical comparison of the patient's symptoms with those of the drug by using a repertory (repertorization). It involves making a choice from among the many different symptoms the patient has presented and establishing a hierarchy on the basis of precision (§ 153, complete symptoms) and ranking value (mind — body — organ), comparing this with the relevant rubrics in the repertory.

The time needed to write everything down can be reduced by using special aids.

1 Value and Significance of Reference Works

Different routes to drug diagnosis were described in the last chapter, pointing out that 'long routes' needed the aid of a repertory and materia medica. In every scientific discipline and any form of serious professional work it is taken for granted that reference works will be consulted, confirming the validity of facts where one feels one cannot entirely trust one's memory. In a complex case it is often impossible to make an immediate decision as to the appropriate drug. Depending on temperament and power of memory, one physician will be able to make a rapid decision whilst another needs to weigh the facts. Basically I have reservations about quick decisions in homoeopathy — good marksmen take careful aim. To paraphrase Lenin, self-confidence is a good thing — self-control is even better.

Finding exactly the right drug means that there has to be close correspondence between the patient's major symptoms and the symptoms obtained in drug tests. Unfortunately we have only one head and the number of symptoms reported by patients and those obtained in drug tests is such that even the best of memories cannot hold them all. None of us can keep in mind more than a rough outline and the basic nature of frequently used drugs, their principal symptoms and modalities. This is nothing to be ashamed of. Hahnemann did of course have profound knowledge of drug symptoms, but even he made up a 'Lexicon of Symptoms' for his personal use.[1]

The number of tested drugs has increased from about 80 in his day to more than 1,000 today. What was right for the master, then, is a genuine necessity for his students. **No responsible homoeopathic physician today can manage without the use of a repertory.** Lack of time in itself makes it impossible to leaf 'blindly' through materia medicas, hoping to find a major symptom listed. We have to resort to a lexicon of symptoms, or repertory as it is now called.

The materia medica describes the signs and symptoms of the drug. The repertory is the index to the materia medica. The materia medica bases itself on the drug, the repertory on the symptoms presented by the patient. The two belong together; both are indispensable tools in drug diagnosis.

In my experience no patient would consider a doctor 'stupid' if he consults a reference work in their presence. Any responsible person will look things up if they feel they cannot entirely trust their memory. Members of the legal profession almost always compare what they know with relevant paragraphs or commentary. Experience has taught us to distrust someone who 'knows it all'. In case of emergency a physician must of course be able to act without first scratching his head three times and solemnly consulting his repertory. When visits have to be made, predominantly in acute cases, the knowledge we carry in our heads will normally suffice. In the consulting room, checking against a repertory in each individual case is a good way of ensuring we do not fall into bad habits.

People who prescribe compound drugs do not need a repertory. They are satisfied once they have set their sights on the pathological diagnosis. To deserve the honourable title of homoeopath, however, it is essential to look for the greatest possible similarity between symptoms.

Such similarity does not call for word-for-word agreement. The meaning of what the patient says must agree with the sensation reported by the person who tested the drug. The symptoms listed in the materia medica derive from many different people involved in drug tests, people speaking different languages and expressing themselves in different ways. It is therefore not surprising if each expresses his subjective sensations in a somewhat different way. The terms used for symptoms are a problem with any repertory. To make up a rubric from a number of individual statements one has to venture to define a common denominator for similar statements. It is important to have a range of similar formulations at hand for every symptom given verbal expression if the exact phrase used by the patient cannot be found in the repertory. For example, sensation of band = as if tied off = like a belt = as if too tight, etc.

Large repertories have the advantage of many cross-references to synonyms. I am always adding new cross-references when consulting the repertory, and this is a useful tip, for it can save much time later on. The greater the number of entries the more useful the index — that is self-understood. A telephone book for example ought to contain every telephone number. From this point of view, the 'lesser' repertories are of more limited value. Yet on the other hand very comprehensive and complete repertories are also more difficult to handle, a disadvantage we have to accept, though it can to some extent be overcome through daily use. One gradually grows so familiar with even the biggest of reference works that its sheer volume ceases to be a problem. Lesser works can cause frustration if the symptom one is looking for is not there.

2 General Description of Various Repertories

A few of the many existing repertories are discussed in more detail below, with selection limited to those most widely used.

Clemens von Boenninghausen, a man taught by Hahnemann himself, was the first to publish a comprehensive repertory. This work holds a special position, and not only from the historical point of view. It has a quality of its own which has set the standard for all other repertories. Hahnemann paid tribute to him in a footnote to § 153 of the *Organon*: 'Excellent work has been done by Regierungsrat (Assistant Secretary in civil service) Baron von Boenninghausen who has compiled a register of characteristic symptoms in his repertory.' This work will be discussed in some detail at a later point.

James Tyler Kent compiled the most comprehensive repertory to date in 1877 (in English). This has been translated into German in two different editions, by G. von Keller and J. Kuenzli von Fimmelsberg and by Erbe. A Synthetic Repertory covering mind and intellect, sexuality, menses and sleep has been published in three languages (English, French, German) by H. Barthel and W. Klunker.

Lesser works worth recommending are Stauffer's *Symptomenverzeichnis* (unfortunately out of print, but sometimes obtainable second-hand) and Dorcsi's *Symptomenverzeichnis*; both are intended as reference works that also convey the characteristic features of the drug one is looking for. Dorcsi has made valuable efforts to integrate homoeopathy into modern medicine in general. His work is well presented and organized and it is handy, providing sufficient information to give orientation.

H. Voisin's *Praktische Homöotherapie* (translated from French) goes entirely its own way. It partly combines the contents of a repertory with a review based on clinical syndromes. A repertory or table is added in the case of certain major syndromes. Some homoeopaths using this work in their surgeries praise it highly, others do not find it helpful. I use it when case-taking has yielded few symptoms and everything is like soft putty. Voisin's book makes it possible to achieve some differentiation, starting from the main complaint, where otherwise one would be limited to organotropic therapy.

3 Design and Contents of Kent's *Repertory*

GENERAL

The fact that Kent's *Repertory* is discussed in particular detail below does not mean that other repertories are considered less important. In my view, everyone should use the tools he finds most useful, depending on his gifts and inclinations. It will be clear from what has been said in the last chapter that different routes are not only possible but are indeed a necessity, depending on the given situation. It is important, however, not to base a philosophy on personal preference and think less of others who use different tools. It is quite unjustifiable to label a colleague who uses Kent's *Repertory* a 'Kentian'. I must admit I do not even know what a 'Kentian' is. Anyone using a telephone book would not be called a 'Telephonian' because of this. Any physician making drug diagnoses according to the Law of Similars is a homoeopath, an honourable title (as Hahnemann called it) which has to be earned over and over again. A comprehensive repertory is a help in this, but certainly no creed.

The chapter headings are on the whole clear, though it should be noted that the chapter entitled 'Generalities' does not comprise a list of 'general symptoms'. It covers many pathological concepts — from abscesses to wounds — and also the nature of the pulse, convulsions, varicose veins, paralysis, weakness, tumours etc.

Within individual chapters, symptoms are arranged on the principle 'from the whole to details, from general to differentiated terms, from the general to the specific'; physically the sequence is head to foot, central to distal, posterior to anterior head. Within rubrics, the sequence is always the same. First comes a comprehensive section listing all the symptoms coming under this heading. This is followed by differentiation into:

1   *Time* of onset or aggravation of a sensation

2   *Concomitants*, modalities, in alphabetical order
3   *Location* — cranial to caudal, proximal to distal
4   *Type* of sensation in alphabetical order
5   *Extending to* — the direction in which pain or sensations radiate.

It is important to learn this sequence by heart, for it will always be repeated; once grasped it facilitates the search.

Unless otherwise stated, details listed under a symptom always refer to aggravation; if a time is given, the symptom occurs or gets worse at that time. The rubric 'Position' in the chapter on 'Sleep' (pp. 1246-7) lists the positions typical for different drugs; no aggravation is involved in this case.

GENERALITIES

Drug diagnosis is based on Hahnemann's view that a lasting cure proceeds from the centre of vital energies to the periphery. When a homoeopathic drug restores order to the central regulation of vital processes, local disease will also be cured, unless the organic lesion has already progressed too far. Phenomena relating to the whole person (general symptoms relating to soul and spirit and to the body and their modalities) are therefore of major significance. It is a disadvantage that these symptoms come in two separate sections, at the beginning (Mind and Vertigo) and end (Sleep, Chill, Fever, Perspiration, Generalities) of Kent's *Repertory*. It is important to note that the general rubrics 'Aversion, food', 'Desires' and 'Thirst' are to be found in the chapter entitled 'Stomach', despite the fact that they do not rank as local symptoms.

The important sphere of sexuality — ranking among general symptoms — is partly included under 'Genitalia, Male' and 'Genitalia, Female' and partly under 'Generalities'.

A number of drugs for chilly patients are listed under 'Heat, vital, lack of' in the chapter on 'Generalities' (pp. 1366-7).

SYMPTOMS RELATING TO SPECIFIC ORGANS
(LOCAL SYMPTOMS)

These are listed in great detail. If a particular differentiation cannot be found, the wider rubric under which the sub-rubric appears may be consulted or synonyms may be looked for. The sequence is always from general to special, from above to below, from occiput to forehead. Within each rubric, the sequence is laterality, time of onset, concomitants, modalities, location, nature of sensations and 'extends to', i.e. the direction in which a sensation radiates (abnormal sensation, pain, numbness etc.)

It sometimes requires practically no effort to find a complete symptom in these differentiated pain rubrics, and this may turn out to be a key symptom.

Example
A patient reports a burning pain in the back of the neck which extends to the occiput. This does not interfere with sleep. Aetiology unknown. Repertorization: pain, burning, cervical region (p. 920), extending to occiput (p. 920), sleep amel. (p. 920). *Calc.* (= *Calcerea carbonica*) is the only drug appearing in all three rubrics. Reference to the materia medica and the subsequent clinical result confirm the accuracy of the drug diagnosis.

GRADING OF DRUGS
Kent graded the drugs listed within a rubric in three categories, to indicate their importance in drug diagnosis.

— **Bold type** — **first grade** — **major importance**
— *Italics* — *second grade* — *medium degree of importance*
— Ordinary type — third grade — lesser degree of importance

Dr Kuenzli von Fimmelsberg uses a reverse order in his German edition of Kent's *Repertory*, calling bold type the third grade and ordinary print the first. This seems very logical, as one would give one point to a drug appearing in ordinary type on repertorization, and three points to one in bold type.

Strictly speaking the use of a points system goes against the homoeopathic principle of differentiating drugs on the basis of the quality of symptoms. If case-taking yields no high-ranking symptoms, however, it may be possible to get an indication of the appropriate drug by collecting 'less brilliant' symptoms and adding them together.

It is important not to take the grading too literally. Kent's system will usually prove reliable, for principal symptoms subject to extensive clinical verification almost always appear in bold type. Polar, alternating and also end effects of the drug are generally shown in italics or ordinary type.

Example
Iodum appears in bold type under Stomach, Appetite, ravenous (p. 478); it is also listed in italics under Stomach, Appetite, wanting (p. 479).

The grades assigned to drugs are helpful when making comparisons between patient and drug. Extreme restlessness shown by the patient must have its match in a drug given the highest grade — in bold type. If a patient says spontaneously and with emphasis that he or she is driven from his or her bed at night by unrest, cannot find rest anywhere, has to get up, the corresponding drug must have the same intense restlessness in bold type (e.g. *Arsenicum, Rhus tox.*)

WORKS COMPLEMENTARY TO KENT'S *REPERTORY*
Ensinger has published a guide to Kent's *Repertory* (in German) which, however, does not offer a complete review.

Flury's *Practical Repertory* is a card repertory (in English, French and German) which forms a bridge between Boenninghausen's emphasis on generalization and the high degree of differentiation to be found in Kent. It contains much useful information relating to symptoms involving the whole person in body and mind.

Barthel and Klunker's Synthetic Repertory (in German) may be used for additional information on mental and mind symptoms, sexuality, menses and sleep.

It would be helpful to have more cross-references in Kent. Eichelberger has issued circulars listing synonyms and alternative expressions (in German). These should be entered in one's repertory. Also, as I said before, it is important always to log new cross-references as they come up in the course of work.

Leers has collected rare symptoms not listed in Kent (in German).

DRUG DIAGNOSIS BY MATCHING SYMPTOMS
In the chapter on Different Methods of Determining the Appropriate Drug, it was said that there are two methods of drug diagnosis:

1   A synthetic view of the clinical picture, comparing this with the drug picture as a whole
2   Analytical evaluation of the patient's individual symptoms, comparing them with similar symptoms from drug tests.

The first, holistic method offers advantages to physicians capable of taking a synthetic view who also know the materia medica extremely well. It can only be used where the material obtained on case-taking comprises idiosyncratic, characteristic symptoms clearly pointing to a particular drug picture.

The second method offers advantages if the case material is fragmentary and does not present a clear picture, so that the drug can only be found by accurate comparison of the list of symptoms. Physicians gifted with a more analytical mind prefer this method. It will give good results even if knowledge of materia medica is limited.

The repertory may be used with both methods, in the first case to look up individual, well differentiated symptoms, in the second case to compare a list of symptoms selected from the case material. If the drug diagnosis seems clear on the whole but doubt attaches to one particular symptom, the repertory will quickly tell us if it belongs to the drug in question. Alternatively, a patient may report a striking symptom we have never heard of. Which drug does it relate to?

Example
I recall my early days in homoeopathy when a mother said her 4-year-old daughter was unable to pass stools if sitting down on the lavatory. If she put her in nappies the young lady would go and stand in a corner and press hard — with immediate success. Stools only when standing. A long search through the English edition of Kent (no translations into German existed at the time) showed 'Constipation, standing, passes stools easier when' on p. 608, with only *Causticum* listed, in bold type.

This was a 'key experience'. It convinced me of the value of a repertory and also of the importance of key symptoms. With key symptoms, complete symptoms or precise general symptoms we do not need a long list, for they tend to be so accurately defined that the rubric usually only contains a small number of drugs. It usually does not require much time to make the final differentiation with the aid of the materia medica and a few further specific questions put to the patient.

The situation is different in a complicated case presenting with a number of incomplete symptoms. Many of these symptoms appear valuable, yet none on its own points to a definite drug. We find a rubric of several drugs for each of these incomplete symptoms in the repertory. Which of these is the one we are looking for?

Each of these symptoms on its own is merely a stone in the mosaic which makes up the whole drug picture. Many stones will gradually let the whole picture emerge to a point where we clearly recognize it. Adding symptom to symptom we group together different parts until we get the whole. An incomplete symptom may not achieve it on its own, but adding many symptoms together we finally determine the drug which is similar and will be able to heal. Adding symptoms together and comparing them in the repertory is a process known as repertorization.

HAHNEMANN'S METHOD
In the introductory memorandum to volume II of his *Materia Medica Pura*, Hahnemann quoted two examples which allow us to look over his shoulder, as it were. This is not only of historical interest, for it demonstrates the essential principle of making a drug diagnosis based on comparison of a number of symptoms:

> W-e, a pale, somewhat debilitated man of 42 whose work always kept him at his desk, complained to me on 27 December 1815 that he had been feeling ill for 5 days.

1   The first evening he felt sick and dizzy for no apparent reason, belching
    frequently
2   the following night (at 2 a.m.) sour vomiting
3   during subsequent nights violent belching
4   at present still troublesome fetid, sour-tasting eructations
5   felt as if food remained in stomach raw and undigested
6   head felt wide, hollow and dark inside and as if sensitive inside
7   least noise upset
8   mild, gentle, long-suffering individual
Comments:

Ad 1) A number of drugs cause dizziness and nausea, among them
Pulsatilla. This also produces vertigo in the evenings, a feature noted with
very few other drugs.

Ad 2) The thorn-apple (*Datura*) and the poison nut (*Nux vomica*) cause
sour and sour-smelling mucilage to be vomited but not, as far as is known,
at night. *Valerian* and Indian cockles (*Cocculus Indicus*) cause vomiting
during the night, but not sour vomiting. Only iron (*Ferrum*) causes
vomiting during the night; it may also provoke sour vomiting, but not
the other symptoms to be taken into account in this case.

Pulsatilla on the other hand causes not only sour vomiting in the
evenings and vomiting during the night altogether, but also the other
symptoms in this case which one would not expect to see with iron.

Ad 3) Night-time eructations are characteristic of *Pulsatilla*.

Ad 4) Stinking, fetid and sour eructations again are characteristic of
Pulsatilla.

Ad 5) Few drugs produce the sensation of undigested food remaining
in the stomach, none of them as completely and strikingly as *Pulsatilla*.

Ad 6) Apart from Ignatius beans (*Ignatia*) — which, however, cannot
provoke the other symptoms we are dealing with— *Pulsatilla* gives rise
to the same condition.

Ad 7) *Pulsatilla* causes this type of thing, and also hypersensitivity of
the other sensory organs, e.g. of vision. Intolerance of noise may also be
found with Indian cockles, Ignatius bean and aconite (*Aconitum*), but
these are not homoeopathic to the other circumstances and have least
of the

Ad 8) mild disposition which, according to the earlier report on *Pulsatilla*,
this plant specifically calls for.

Nothing therefore would cure this patient more easily, with greater
certainty and more lastingly than *Pulsatilla* which in this case was
homoeopathic. He was given this immediately, but in view of his debilitated
condition in greatly reduced dosage, i.e. half a drop of a quadrillionth
of a strong solution of *Pulsatilla*. This happened towards evening.

The following day he was relieved of all his symptoms, his digestion
had been restored to normal, and he continued well and in good health,
as I heard from him a week later.

The study of such a minor case of illness and the selection of the appropriate agent is very quickly done by someone with a moderate degree of experience who has the symptoms of the drug partly in mind and partly knows where to find them quickly; to put it all down in writing, however, listing points in favour and against (it only takes a few moments to survey these in one's mind) makes for tiresome verbosity, as may be seen.

For one's personal use in practice, it is merely necessary to jot down for every individual symptom the drugs which produce as nearly as possible the same symptom (just a few letters for each, e.g. *Ferr., Chin., Rheum, Puls.*), and to keep in mind the conditions under which they do so, as this influences the choice. One continues like this for every other symptom — which drug causes each of them — to conclude from the resulting list which of the drugs is able to cover most of the symptoms under consideration homoeopathically, above all the most peculiar and characteristic symptoms. This, then, is the drug we are looking for.

Drug diagnosis based on comparison of symptoms therefore requires the physician partly to have the drug symptoms in his head and partly to know where to find them.

This is the point where Hahnemann's followers took over. Ways had to be found to allow symptoms to be 'quickly found' in practice. The general review of different repertories has already shown that different methods may be used. This gives every homoeopathic physician the freedom to use his own method of finding symptoms quickly.

VON BOENNINGHAUSEN AS THE INVENTOR OF REPERTORIZATION

The particular importance of von Boenninghausen's repertory has already been mentioned. His method of selecting symptoms for drug diagnosis merits more detailed attention.

von Boenninghausen's painstaking, conscientious efforts led to the compilation of individual drug symptoms. His achievement goes beyond mere industriousness, however, for he did not get bogged down in detail and was consistent in the way he continued Hahnemann's work. Thanks to him, the law of similars has become a practical proposition even in complex cases lacking immediate clarity.

von Boenninghausen clearly understood that comprehensive case-taking involving a multiplicity of symptoms becomes possible only if symptoms are organized and graded in a meaningful way.

It is not possible to compare every minor, incomplete symptom with the symptomatology of a drug. The whole ranks above its parts.

von Boenninghausen therefore favoured symptoms which provide specific information relating to the sensations and modalities of the whole person. General symptoms relating to body, soul and spirit determine the drug diagnosis. He thus implemented the concepts put forward by Hahnemann that:

> All parts of the organism are thus intimately bound up with each other, forming an indivisible whole in our perceptions and functionally (*Organon* § 189). Genuine treatment applied by a physician to a disorder which has arisen in external parts of the body should therefore be directed to the whole, to the annihilation and cure of the general malady . . . , if it is to be effective, reliable, thorough and helpful. (*Organon* § 190)

von Boenninghausen combines a number of individual symptoms in a general symptom if they are similar in nature regarding modality and sensation.

Example

A patient complains 1) that for some time she has had lancinating pains in the knee joint when walking. Fango packs had if anything made it worse. 2) For the last few days she had had a cough with sharp pains in the chest, particularly on taking a deep breath. The cough was worse on entering a warm room. 3) When she had her period she would experience a sharp pain in the right ovary if she took the stairs quickly.

The same sensation, a sharp pain, occurred in all these locations, also the same modality, worse on movement (walking, taking a deep breath, stairs), worse from heat (packs, warm room).

Three separate symptoms have thus become a valuable general symptom, easy to find in the repertory and also easily recognizable: *Bryonia*.

By establishing rank and order and by generalization, von Boenninghausen concentrated the totality of symptoms (the mass) into the sum and essence of symptoms, a qualitative aspect. He achieved the implementation of Hahnemann's dictum that particular value should attach to peculiar and characteristic signs and symptoms.

This made him the initiator of a clear, repeatable scientific method of drug diagnosis. von Boenninghausen has given us the key to meaningful use of the repertory: **We should never be slaves to detail, losing ourselves in the multiplicity of individual symptoms.** The use of a repertory should not end up as a caricature of itself — leafing through the book for hours, searching here and there, and making the hunt for unusual symptoms an end in itself. A repertory is an aid and should remain so. It does not influence the basic principles of drug diagnosis but merely jogs our memory, making it possible to use the rich abundance of drug symptoms in making the drug diagnosis in a particular case. People who really know the materia medica find themselves surprised over and over again at the tremendous variety it offers. The real experts acknowledge, in all humility, that one's memory needs the support of a repertory of symptoms. It is difficult to understand why colourful drug pictures are narrowed down over the years to woodcuts printed in black and white and committed to memory as such. There is the cliché for example of the blue-eyed, blonde, gentle, weepy *Pulsatilla* female; yet people often forget that this gentle drug presents with burning pains in many areas. As an index to a comprehensive materia medica, the repertory can convey to us a vast symptomatology, overcoming such clichés. Comparing repertory and materia medica and vice versa we come to perceive the full reality of the drug, and as a result our treatment becomes more effective.

KENT — MASTER OF DETAIL

Kent's unique achievement has been to make the great abundance of materia medica accessible to us in his *Repertory*. He built on the foundations laid by von Boenninghausen. The particular characteristic of Kent's work is his propensity for detail. This also places drug symptoms in their original context.

Example
Under 'Cough, Raised, child must be, gets blue in face, cannot exhale — *Mephitis*.' (p. 801)

Accuracy concerning individual symptoms was his special interest. Exaggerating to make the point, we might say that von Boenninghausen generalized whilst Kent differentiated.

In stark contrast these approaches may seem contradictory. In practice we need both individual detail and generalities for repertorization.

Hahnemann's *Organon* states that the essential in making the drug diagnosis is that 'in choosing the homoeopathic drug specific to the case, particular and almost exclusive attention must be given to the more remarkable, peculiar, unusual and singular (characteristic) signs and symptoms.' (§ 153). Remarkable, peculiar and unusual features usually attach to individual symptoms. Characteristic features tend to go beyond individual symptoms and relate to the whole person.

It is peculiar, for instance, for a patient to say that his knees are cold in bed at night (*Phosphorus, Sepia*). If on the other hand he complains of feeling cold through and through, being unable to get warm even in summer, this lack of vital heat (p. 1367) is characteristic of that person.

The peculiar nature of the whole person *and* the unique features of individual symptoms and signs have to be recognized.

Hahnemann almost always used very exact formulations, but unfortunately we tend to read past them too quickly. Section 153 of the *Organon* — the pivot of the drug diagnosis — lists important symptoms in two categories, on the one hand those that are remarkable, peculiar and unusual, on the other hand those that are singular or characteristic. The two groups are linked with an 'and'. Until I came to grasp the significance of this 'and', I used to find myself stumbling among the different suggestions made as to how the appropriate drug was to be found; they made me feel insecure. Advice on the method of repertorization ranges from one extreme of considering individual symptoms in minute detail (remarkable, peculiar) to the other of almost exclusively depending on general symptoms (singular, characteristic). Some authors advise against the utilization of symptoms deriving from the sphere of the principal complaint, paying particular attention to general symptoms instead.

Hahnemann's 'and' is the link between the extremes advocated by his successors, telling us to make use of remarkable and peculiar as well as general and characteristic symptoms.

5 Method of Repertorization
Treatment must always be preceded by diagnosis. Every drug diagnosis is preceded by high-quality case-taking. The more confusing the case, the more thorough must our case-taking be. This is something to be stressed over and over again.

Repertorization requires a written record of the material obtained on case-taking. The totality of symptoms must be determined (see chapter on Case-Taking). This 'raw material' consisting of clinical diagnostic concepts, signs, symptoms and biographical data then needs to be sifted and organized. The goal of the organizing process is to derive the sum and essence of symptoms from the total material, to separate the essential elements out from the multiplicity. This brings us to a crucial question: Which of the symptoms should one select? The question has two sides to it and requires an answer from the negative as well as the positive point of view.

SELECTION, ORGANIZATION AND EVALUATION OF SYMPTOMS
It will no doubt be obvious from what has gone before that indefinite and obvious symptoms are left aside. We do not pick indifferent players for the national team.

> More general and indefinite symptoms such as lack of appetite, headache, tiredness, restless sleep, malaise etc. merit little attention, seeing they are

general, unless they are more specifically defined; such general symptoms are seen in almost every case of illness and with almost every drug. (*Organon* § 153)

Anything which serves to demonstrate individual differences is part of the sum and essence — every detail in the picture is not.

For practical reasons alone, it is not possible to utilize every symptom obtained by extensive case-taking, look it up in the repertory and write down the drugs listed in the rubric. It would take hour upon hour — writing things down, looking them up, writing, looking up — and the outcome would be of little value in determining therapy. The method could be compared to someone wishing to describe an apple tree and going into the minutest detail of every single apple — its colour, size, shape, any marks, worms etc., then going on to examine every twig and every leaf in great detail. The characteristic nature of the tree and the sun and essence of its features (root, trunk, crown) would be completely lost in the mass of detail.

We tend to baulk at the seeming paradox of first of all going to great lengths to collect the totality of symptoms and then throwing a lot of the material out again. The paradox is only a seeming one, however, for it is impossible to determine whilst we are case-taking which group of symptoms will serve to indicate the appropriate drug. Archaeologists also record every single stone they unearth and its position until it becomes clear that the stones lying around in various places are what is left of a wall, say. Following this realization, individual stones become part of the wider concept 'wall'.

In positive terms, the question as to which symptoms to select may be answered as follows:

Select the symptoms which characterize the whole person and also symptoms which are remarkable, peculiar and unusual in the concrete case you are dealing with.

It will depend on the case material collected in each individual case as to which aspect emerges more clearly in the symptomatology. The multiplicity of pathological processes forces us to differentiate in the selection of symptoms. In same cases patients give a fairly precise description of one or two peculiar symptoms, and these may even be given as complete symptoms, with aetiology, location, type, modality and concomitants. In other cases, particularly with chronic conditions that have persisted for a long time, individual symptoms are mere fragments or purely pathognomic and there is nothing outstanding. On the other hand we often find highly characteristic symptoms in such cases if we go into the whole mental and physical make-up of the person.

In a third group of patients an unusual or even paradox symptom may present itself as the 'distinguishing mark of the drug' (von Keller); a clearly defined sensation (as if the heart would stop); a remarkable modality (everything worse on movement); an unexpected mental reaction (furious if consoled) or a peculiar location (headache beneath roof of orbit). Each of these can take us close to the drug we are looking for.

Ideally case-taking yields a number of symptoms of real value both individually and in relation to the whole. If this ideal cannot be achieved we must confine ourselves to the area for which precise symptoms are available. Potential choice does of course depend on a certain volume of material being available.

Repertorization is based on selected symptoms. Anything indefinite or expected is eliminated and so are minor details which do not characterize the patient or a drug. The sum and essence of symptoms is derived from the totality.

The sum and essence of symptoms includes:
— **anything characteristic of the whole person, his or her peculiar character relating to soul and spirit and also to the physical organization (general symptoms);**
— **organ-specific and local symptoms in their particular individual form if precisely defined, remarkable, peculiar and singular (specifically individual local symptoms).**

It is the case material which in the individual case determines whether the emphasis is more on general characteristics or on particular and peculiar symptoms. Rigid adherence to a system would fail to allow for the multiplicity of pathological processes. The following examples may show how in one case the principal complaint leads us to the drug because it has a particular individual character, whilst in other cases characteristic general symptoms play the leading role. An optimum may be achieved where it is possible to choose between a number of high-quality symptoms from both spheres.

Having selected our symptoms from the total case material we proceed to the second step which is to organize the symptoms and to grade them.

The best system for establishing order among the many symptoms is according to whether they relate to body and soul as a whole or whether they are particular (local symptoms). Efforts should be made to construct a whole symptom out of the fragments which on case-taking appear here and there (aetiology, location, type, modality, concomitants).

The ranking order attached to symptoms depends on the quality of their description — whether they are precise and/or complete and where they come in the hierarchic sequence of mind, intellect, body, organ.

Once a certain experience has been gained it is possible to combine the three stages of selection, organization and valuation. A useful tip is first of all to underline in red in your notes or on the questionnaire all major symptoms relating to the whole individual (general symptoms relating to body and soul). A blue pencil may then be used to underline all important local symptoms which have been accurately defined. One would of course be on the look-out all the time for at least one complete symptom with its concomitants. This completes selection, organization and valuation. The underlining marks out the symptoms we include and indicates their category. Having underlined the symptoms in this way, it is important to check and see if the selection stands up to critical assessment.

It is important to be self-critical. This is analogous to setting out a mathematical problem, which must be done exactly right if the correct solution is to be found. The selection and organization of symptoms must be in full accord with the reality of the patient if drug diagnosis is to lead to the simile. The symptoms assigned the highest rank because they relate to the whole person must be really outstanding in the patient. They must really have almost forced themselves on us during case-taking. Symptoms relating to soul and spirit, for instance, tend to lack precision in many cases. One has to know a person for a time before their nature really emerges. A patient needs to develop confidence in his or her physician before 'deeper' things can be mentioned. Unfortunately many physicians do not have the greatest of gifts or the training to enable them to see behind the facade. Not every patient is so much of an exhibitionist that he will bare his soul unasked. von Boenninghausen was more modest than Kent, placing 'mind' symptoms at the end of his list and using them to confirm or eliminate the drug he had chosen. His advice was to read the mental symptoms up in the materia medica and make a careful comparison. He is very much in agreement with Hahnemann in this. In the examples Hahnemann gave of making a drug diagnosis, 'mind' symptoms were listed at the end and used to confirm the choice of drug.

RANKING ORDER OF SYMPTOMS

The criteria for selecting symptoms on which to base the drug diagnosis have already been discussed in Chapter VI. They are important, however, and we shall therefore recapitulate the major points. It is essential for repertorization to establish a sequence of symptoms for every individual case. The sequence is determined by general rules which have to be adapted to individual circumstances.

The quality of a symptom depends on two factors: its precision and a high rank in the scale of personal validity. Symptoms have to be seen through, as it were, from both points of view to determine their quality. This might be put in a formula: precision x rank = quality. There are three possible combinations:

Table 6: Evaluation of Case Material

Symptoms	Aspects determining precision	Ranking order	Quality
Someone looking over shoulder	Remarkable, peculiar, clearly described intense experience, persisting a long time	Mind symptom, illusion	very good
'As if someone present'	highly peculiar	'As if' symptom Aetiology of her fear	very good
Felt very well at seaside	Emphatically put and a definite experience. Persisting for a long time	General physical symptom	valuable
Menses: interval short	Not very accurate, — no remarkable abnormality in duration and consistency of menses	General physical symptom	good
Acne	Typical form w. little precision. Acne better at seaside is not really remarkable as acne generally better in summer and in open air	Principal complaint: local pathognomic sign lacking differentiation	limited
Perspires easily on exertion	Not remarkable in corpulent subjects	General physical symptom	limited
Afraid in dark, afraid in the evenings	Not unusual, many people have it. Not existential fear as described. Patient more inclined to consider it funny; it annoys her.	Mind symptom with modality	reasonably good

1　A high-ranking symptom, e.g. a 'mind' symptom which lacks precision and completeness and perhaps has been getting less marked recently will be poorer in quality than it should normally be because of this lack of precision.

2　High quality attaches to a remarkable and complete local symptom with unusual concomitants that has been spontaneously mentioned by the patient and strongly felt by him or her, having persisted for a long time or been growing more marked. Here particular precision elevates the usually low ranking order of a local symptom.

3　A combination of precision and high personal validity results in optimum quality and the almost mathematical certainty that a cure will be achieved.

Example

A tall, robust and also plump lady complained primarily of severe acne. Locally there was nothing outstanding — a case of acne like many others. Her spontaneous report and specific questions also yielded no differentiating data. Yet when she noted that my indirect questions expressed an interest in herself she said quite spontaneously: 'It is odd, I have felt rather annoyed with myself for some time now because I get scared driving the car at night, when it is dark; it feels as if someone were looking over my shoulder, as if there were someone present.' Further questioning revealed that menses tended to be early, she perspired quickly on physical exertion, e.g. if active in sport; felt very well by the seaside, and her acne had been much better when she had been there in the summer.

Table 7: Repertorization of the Case (Kent's *Repertory*)

Someone looking over shoulder (Delusions, people, behind her, someone is) p. 30	Feels very well at seaside (Air, seashore amel.) p. 1344 Med. only	Menses, interval too short, too early p. 726	Acne p. 366	Pimples, face p. 1315	Perspires on least exertion p. 1297	Afraid in dark, in the evenings pp. 42, 43
Anacard. Brom. Calc. Casc. Cench. Crot.c. Lach. Med. Ruta Staph. Sil.	Brom. Med. Nat.mur.	*Anacard.* Brom. **Calc.** Lach. Ruta Staph. Sil.	Brom. not mentioned	Brom.	Brom.	Brom.

The symptoms I selected have been arranged in order of quality in the table. Beginners may be surprised to find that the principal complaint, the clinical diagnosis of 'acne', appears fairly late in the list. It should also be noted that 'fear', a high-ranking mental symptom, has been put last because the fear was not very marked in this case.

Bromium occurs in the greatest number of rubrics and particularly also in those ranking highest. Reference to the materia medica, e.g. to Boericke, confirmed similarity to the whole person and the principal complaint. Kent unfortunately does not list *Bromium* under 'acne', though it may be found under 'pimples' and 'boils'. Bromine acne is, however, well known from toxicology. Voison (1969) lists *Bromium* as the drug of choice for acne in corpulent subjects — confirming typological agreement in the case under discussion.

Drug diagnosis must start from the whole. The direction of cure is from the centre outwards. If one wishes to achieve a cure there is little point in basing drug diagnosis on local symptoms and local modalities and ignoring the fact that there is no agreement at the level of totality. Such a method would only achieve temporary palliation. The cure proceeds from within outwards, and the symptoms which determine the choice of drug must reflect this inner disruption of vital energy. The disruption of vital energy is often well represented in 'general' symptoms. When they are of high quality, these symptoms rank above all others.

Arrange all symptoms according to their quality. The precision and intensity of statements will be more apparent in case-material obtained personally than with questionnaires. With this proviso regarding rank and quality, symptoms may be arranged in sequence more or less as follows:

1 Complete symptoms meeting the conditions laid down in § 153
2 Remarkable mental symptoms, ideally with modality
3 Well-marked general physical symptoms (general symptoms and modalities)
4 Convincing aetiological symptoms
5 Unusual concomitants
6 Peculiar and striking local symptoms.

PUTTING IT DOWN ON PAPER

The symptoms which have been selected are arranged according to quality. I like to use a sheet of A4 paper, taking it sideways. It is also possible to use preprinted repertorization sheets (e.g. the one by Voegeli). Leers's punched-card system is useful if one wants to save time.

The above case may serve as an example to give us a feeling for the quality of symptoms. Repertorization is anything but sheer mechanical comparison of a number of symptoms. In every single case, the symptomatology has to be assessed for quality.

The search should be a systematic one, to avoid the useless waste of time.

First point to be considered: Where does this symptom belong? Where do I find it? Is it a sensation; a modality relating to the whole person; a general mental or physical symptom? Or is the element under consideration only a partial aspect of the symptomatology — is the sensation, the pain, linked to a location; is the nature or time-relation of the sensation given (e.g. on waking in the mornings)?

Second point to be considered: Is the symptom merely a fragment or is it almost complete?

Consideration of these two points shows whether the search should start with one of the large rubrics or whether there is hope of finding a smaller, more precise, sub-rubric. Kent's *Repertory* offers the advantage of having both, so that it is possible to adapt, depending on the case material. Several large rubrics lacking sharp definition or one small but very precise rubric will in the end achieve the same.

Drug diagnosis based on large rubrics will lead to major drugs (polychrests), sometimes excluding minor, less well tested, drugs. This is an obvious disadvantage to working with large rubrics. If on the other hand a smaller sub-rubric is chosen, we must make sure that the sum and essence of symptoms, the whole person, is properly matched. It is necessary to guard against either of these dangers by consulting the materia medica. Comparison with a large materia medica (e.g. Hering, Allen)[1] often shows that lesser drugs are cut down to almost nothing in the smaller materia medicas, reduced to an organotropic shadow. It is therefore important to check against a materia medica particularly if lesser drugs are chosen; the polychrests are reasonably well known to most of us.

Repertorization may proceed from 'above', starting with large general rubrics, or from 'below', using highly differentiated individual symptoms, though the latter must be very marked.

In the repertory, we look for the expression which most clearly resembles the words used by the patient.

Example
A patient says: 'I dream with my eyes open.' The phrase corresponding most closely to this in Kent is 'Dreams, awake, while' on p. 1236.

Many patients refer to their pain as 'throbbing'. The nearest to this in Kent is '(Head) pulsating (p. 223) or hammering', depending on the intensity of the throbbing sensation.

The list is easier to survey if the same drugs are written in the same line and linked by lines drawn between them.

The different grades are best indicated by underlining:
— doubly underlined = first (highest) grade
— singly underlined = second (middle) grade
— not underlined = 3rd (lowest) grade.

This gives a clear picture, making it immediately obvious which are the dominant drugs in the list.

The rubric must correspond exactly to the statement made by the patient. 'Desire for open air' (p. 1343) means that the patient has a real longing for the open air and cannot live without fresh air. 'Open air amel.' (p. 1344) means that his symptoms are better. Distinction has to be made between 'Motion agg.' (p. 1374) and 'Motion, aversion to' (p. 1375); the former means that there is a physical sensation of symptoms being worse on movement, whilst the latter gives expression more to psychological motivation.

Fear and anxiety on the other hand cannot always be cleanly separated. In this case it is best to look under both terms. When someone tells us that they feel nervous when walking, the closest rubrics are 'Anxiety, walking, while'(p. 9) and 'Fear, walking, while' (p. 47). Depending on the situation, it may be best to combine the two rubrics or to choose one of them.

These few examples may encourage the reader to reflect and to talk to his or her patients. It is often surprising how accurately patients will describe their sensations once they feel we are really interested in them as a person.

ELIMINATING SYMPTOMS
If case-taking has resulted in good quality general symptoms relating to large rubrics with many drugs in the repertory, 'eliminating symptoms' are used first to reduce the amount of writing needed. As far as I know the idea came from Drs Margaret Tyler and John Weir. [2]

Example (see Table 8)
A patient complained that for 3 months he felt utterly confused in the mornings. He compared this to 'two large glasses of wine too many'. Asked about the time, 'in the mornings' being somewhat vague, he said that the condition persisted until about 10 a.m. It made no difference whether he stayed in bed or got up. It was, however, worse for a while after breakfast.

The following rubrics may be considered: ('Confusion of mind, morning' (p. 13), 'intoxicated, as if' (p. 15), 'intoxicated, as after being (p. 15), 'eating, after' (p. 15). Writing out all the drugs listed under those symptoms would take quite a lot of time. The first rubric alone comprises 103 drugs. It was possible to reduce the amount of work considerably in this case, for case-taking had shown the patient to be very chilly; he caught cold easily and did not tolerate cold air. The drug therefore had to be a 'cold' one. The rubric 'Heat, vital, lack of' has all the 'Icemen' (p. 1366). 'Coldness' was a consistent peculiar characteristic of this patient and it was therefore possible to eliminate all drugs which did not come under that rubric. I have written the drugs of this rubric on a piece of card. If I get such a case I put the card at the beginning of the list of symptoms and only take the drugs which are listed on it from any further rubric I consult, eliminating all 'hot' drugs. This reduces the amount of writing by about half. One uses grade one symptoms for this, and they must really be marked.

The opposite of the 'Icemen' are the 'Furnaces', people who are hot, with an excess of heat. They will say: 'I am always too hot; I don't like summer at all.' We can often recognize them from the clothes they wear, for even when winter is at its hardest they will be only lightly clad. A patient talking about her husband said:

> Even in winter he will sit in the living room in his pyjamas in the mornings, calmly reading his paper; it does not even bother him if I open all the windows to air the room. Long underpants are for sissies in his view. He does not need a hat, nor a winter coat. He never goes to Italy or Spain for his holidays, saying he's not a southerner. Last year I had to go to the North Cape with him.

Such descriptions really bring people to life. For a drug diagnosis and particularly for determining eliminating symptoms, this living overall impression must be channelled into the terms we find in the repertory: 'Warm agg.' (p. 1412); 'Warm air agg.' (p. 1412); 'Warm wraps agg.' (p. 1412); 'Warm room agg.' (p. 1413); 'Warm wet weather agg.' (p. 1413). These symptoms may be used to eliminate 'cold' drugs and consequently large rubrics as a preliminary step in repertorization. Again I use a piece of card on which all drugs showing overall aggravation from heat or warmth (p. 1412) are listed. The statement 'warm agg.' requires more careful differentiation than is needed with chilly patients. The group includes patients who feel really unwell in warm wet weather; others do not like warm clothes, and sometimes problems arise from being in a hot or warm room. The rubrics listed above refer to these differences. **These peculiar reactions can only be used as eliminating symptoms if the patient is really emphatic about them.**

It is important to note that some patients are sensitive to both cold and hot conditions. *Mercurius* for instance tends to feel hot if acutely ill and to be aggravated by heat, yet a *Mercurius* patient suffering from chronic illness tends to react unfavourably to cold. Extremes of temperature are not well tolerated by *Mercurius, Cinnabaris, Ipecacuanha* and *Natrum carb.* If a patient says he feels very chilly, we must ask further questions to make sure he is not merely considering his present, chilly, condition, failing to remember the opposite phase. *Iodum* is generally a very 'hot' drug, but emaciated *Iodum* patients may be

Table 8

Heat. vital, lack of p. 1367 Grade 1 drugs only	Consolation agg. p. 16	Confusion morning p. 13	-intoxicated as if p. 15	-intoxicated as after being p. 15	-eating, after p.15
Aran.					
Ars.	*Ars.*	Ars.			
Bar-c.					
Calc.	Calc.	*Calc.*			Calc.
Calc-ar.					
Calc-p.	*Calc-p.*				
Camph.					
Carb-an.					
Caust.					
Cist.					
Crot-c.					
Dulc.					
Ferr.					
Graph.					
Helo.					
Hep.					
Kali-ar.					
Kali-bi.					
Kali-c.	Kali-c.	Kali-c.		Kali-c.	
Kali-p.					
Led.					
Mag-p.					
Nit-ac.	Nit-ac.				
Nux-v.	Nux-v.	Nux-v.	Nux-v.	*Nux-v.*	*Nux-v.*
Ph-ac.					
Phos.					
Psor.					
Pyrog.					
Rhus-t.					
Sil.					

chilly in the final stage. *Sulphur* shows a similar reaction. Young sulphurics tend to be heated, but in old age *Sulphur* is often chilly.

Apart from reactions to heat and cold, the attitude to consolation may be used as an eliminating symptom. Most people respond positively to consolation, kind words, and sympathy with their problems — unless it is done crudely or awkwardly. There are others, however, who refuse consolation (Consolation agg. p. 16), and others again react with anger (p. 3). These symptoms are so striking that the 'consolation test' can be used to eliminate or confirm a large number of drugs. *Phos.* for instance has 'better from consolation', *Arsenicum* refuses it. Kent only lists *Pulsatilla* under 'Consolation amel.', but it is necessary to take a wider view. In the case of *Pulsatilla* it is remarkable how quickly consolation improves the condition — a minute ago there were tears, now the sun is shining again.

Example
In the case described above, it was my great good fortune that apart from marked chilliness the patient also showed marked aversion to consolation. His actual words were: 'What's the good of consolation, such a silly to-do only gets on my nerves.'

Table 8 shows how little writing remained to be done. The first column was provided by the piece of card on which the 'cold' drugs were already listed. Only those 'cold' drugs were then put down in the column headed 'consolation agg.' This left only 4 out of 103 drugs for the column headed 'Confusion, morning', all others having been excluded on the basis of the two elimination symptoms used in the first two columns.

The final authority is the materia medica. The repertory has served as an index to the materia medica, pointing the way to particular drug. **Analytical comparison of individual symptoms finally ends again with a synthetic overview of the whole drug picture.** Now we have to establish if the patient as a unique individual really resembles the drug in question, whether it matches him overall. If there is no such correspondence between patient and drug, we have gone wrong in our analysis of the case material.

6　Time-Savers
Repertorization is time-consuming. Writing down the lists of drugs is laborious. To the best of my knowledge it was Boger who first thought of using a punched-card index to save work. Leers later published a good punched-card index in German.

Card repertories prove real time-savers if large rubrics are used, i.e. symptoms common to many drugs. Minor unusual symptoms found only with two or three drugs are just as quickly written out from the book. It is evident, therefore, that card repertorization has its uses mainly for large general rubrics. It makes it possible to reduce a long list of drugs to just a few polychrests. Finer differentiation on the basis of lesser but peculiar symptoms and modalities can then be based on this group of related drugs. The method is highly effective in chronic cases with clearly defined general symptoms. Acute conditions with high-ranking remarkable symptoms are just as quickly repertorized by the traditional book method. Leers' card system is on the whole based on Kent's *Repertory*. Using the card system and the book in combination thus offers the best potential. Leers is constantly adding to the number of punched cards, and his method has served to extend the repertorization technique. We are greatly indebted to him, because his work has made it possible to achieve two basically irreconcilable aims — to save time and improve quality.

The latest fashion is computer-based repertorization — and this certainly does not come cheap. Still, if one considers the prices of the equipment — most of it useless — used in modern surgeries, we can perhaps say that it is only right for us to have the best of tools as well. Time will tell if the method is really effective. The best of computers cannot provide more information than has been input by human minds.

There is one major objection to which some thought should be given.

Comparison is made between *qualitative* aspects, and any form of quantification, any totting up, is apt to do more harm than good. It has been the experience with modern technology that we succumb only too easily to the machines, becoming their willing slaves. The question is — Who's to be master?

When a mathematical equation has been wrongly set out, the result is no more accurate whichever method of calculation we use. This also applies to any method of drug diagnosis, including repertorization. It is essential always to be very much awake and adaptable, to have professional skill, the ability to feel one's way into the personal situation of the patient, and the desire to do good homoeopathic work.

7 Summary
It is not always possible to make a differentiated drug diagnosis based on the law of similars without recourse to reference works. The sheer volume of data goes beyond the capacity of even the best of human memories. The materia medica and repertory are valuable aids if used together. Hahnemann himself compiled a 'Lexicon of Symptoms' for his personal use, to make it possible to 'find symptoms quickly'. von Boenninghausen took the work of his teacher further and published

the first large repertory. This is remarkable not only for the amount of work that has gone into it but also because it established a technique of finding the simile by comparing symptoms relating to the patient as a whole with the symptoms due to drug action which are listed in the repertory. Later authors, above all Kent, used von Boenninghausen's work as the basis for their own work. Kent's pariticular contribution has been the more subtle differentiation of local symptoms. Kent's *Repertory* is now used all over the world.

Repertorization depends on good quality case-taking and a written record being made of the symptomatology. Evaluation and grading reduces the many symptoms forming the totality to a small number representing the sum and essence. These high-quality symptoms are looked up in the repertory, writing down the drugs listed in the relevant rubrics. Two or three drugs will usually dominate the picture. These are then looked up in the materia medica before the final decision is made as to which drug corresponds to the sick individual as a whole.

The analytical process of drug diagnosis based on a list of symptoms is finally verified by comparison with the drug picture, taking a synthetic approach.

The amount of writing involved can be time-consuming, but it is possible to save time by using a punched-card index (Boger, Leers). Repertorization technique is an aid, not an aim in itself.

The technique has to be adapted to the individual needs of physician and patient. Drug diagnosis may in some cases be based on the combination of several large rubrics in the repertory relating to high-quality symptoms involving the whole person. In other cases, where individual symptoms are very accurately defined and differentiated, it may be possible to combine these in a complete symptom which then serves as a key symptom leading us directly to the appropriate drug.

With either method it is important to judge the quality of a symptom by considering both the degree of accuracy of definition and the position in the hierarchy of the person.

The route chosen, from whole to detail or from detail to whole, is confirmed by consulting the materia medica. Prescriptions based entirely on individual symptoms can only achieve palliation. The particular value of repertorization is that it makes it possible to find a common denominator for local and general symptoms. The drug which is finally chosen must correspond to the sick individual with regard to his overall reactivity.

Repertorization is a technical aid offering an extended potential of finding the appropriate drug. **It should never block our view of the sick individual.**

---

[1] T. F. Allen's 12-vol. *Encyclopaedia of Pure Materia Medica* and C. Hering's 10-vol. work contain a rich abundance of symptoms covering all drugs tested up to that time. If a decision has to be made between them, I would advice Hering. It is better set out and printed and well-proven symptoms are more clearly emphasized. Both works are obtainable at a reasonable price from India.

[2] Tyler M, & Weir J. Repertorizing. *Br Hom J* 1983; **72**: 199ff.

8

PRINCIPLES GOVERNING CHOICE OF POTENCY, DOSE, DURATION AND REPETITION OF DRUG THERAPY

Selection of the appropriate drug is the first prerequisite if treatment is to be successful.

The choice of potency and dose should correspond to the patient's reactivity at the given time. It does, however, also depend on the activity of the drug in the unpotentized state.

The dose — i.e. the 'amount' of substance or energy — needs to be in line with the laws of stimulant therapy: the greater the irritant effect the smaller the dose, the more inert the substance the greater the dose. In homoeopathy, 'dose' means the number of drops or tablets.

When substances are highly attenuated, the dose is not determined in milligrams, but on the basis of the alterative energy eliciting a noticeable reaction. The reaction observed in the patient also suggests if and when medication is to be repeated.

The homoeopathic drug has been selected by the 'long or short route'. The materia medica has been consulted to ensure that the drug really matches the overall reactivity of the patient.

This is the point when the final decisions have to be made concerning the prescription. The points to be considered are:
1   potency
2   dose
3   repetition of dose.

1 Potency
Hahnemann initially used unpotentized drugs, yet his treatment was homoeopathic. The point at issue is agreement between the drug picture and the individual picture presented by the patient. Adapting the potency to the patient's 'sensitivity' is very important but only ranks second. A cure can be achieved with low ($\emptyset$ — 6x), medium (12x — 21x) and high (30c and above) potencies. The choice of potency is no

confession of faith. It bases on unbiased observation and on experience gained by generations of physicians.

It is known from toxicology that massive poisoning causes destructive tissue changes; chronic poisoning with smaller doses leads to functional disorders. The subtle toxicology of homoeopathic drug tests yields mental symptoms.

Voisin in particular has assessed drug test records to determine the interval after which particular reactions occur in the test subjects given particular potencies. He was able to confirm the same sequence: low potencies are organotropic, medium potencies influence function, higher potencies the psyche.

This scale provides the basis for the first principle governing the choice of potency:

> low   in organic disease
> medium   for functional disorders
> high   for mental symptoms.

The second principle bases on the medicinal quality of the drug in its unpotentized state. Quite a few people have gold in their mouths as prosthetic material. Does this have medicinal actions? Gold and other insoluble substances only become medicinal on potentization. The medicinal action starts when colloidal solubility is reached, at about 8x. In the case of gold, this would be the lowest potency at which an effect may be expected (bioavailability). The terms 'high', 'medium' and 'low' are indeed relative. The standard to be applied is activity in organisms subject to pathological change.

Medicinal herbs containing highly toxic alkaloids (e.g. aconitine in the case of aconite, the dose lethal to man being 4-6mg) are too aggressive if used in low potencies. The curative, alterative phase starts only from the medium potency range, about the 12x.

Mercury given in form of *Mercurius sol.* has toxic effects on the intestinal and oral flora up to the 6x. This explains why low potencies of *Mercurius* can have a bacteriostatic effect on the surface of the tonsils and provoke immune reactions if not properly homoeopathic.

The poison of the bushmaster snake (*Lachesis muta*) contains haemolytic enzymes. Low potencies may provoke haemorrhages if there is a disposition; I have observed epistaxis in patients given the 8x. The potency chosen to heal homoeopathically should therefore be above that level. Homoeopathy calls for individual tailoring even when it comes to choosing the potency.

The second principle may be formulated as follows:

The lowest medicinal potency for drugs with practically no medicinal properties in the unpotentized state usually corresponds to their colloidal solubility (from about 8x upwards). Highly toxic drugs only show alterative properties above their 'aggressive' range (from about the 12x upwards).

The third principle derives from the observation that there is considerable variation in individual reactivity. The phenomenon of allergic or hyperergic reactions to minimal stimulus serves to indicate that many patients are highly sensitive to stimulus. Individual sensitivity is very much greater in subjects with vegetative imbalance than in those with stable sympathicotonic or parasympathicotonic regulation. The first hints of vegetative instability are obtainable by observing pupillary reactions. This does of course presuppose that there is no neurological or local ophthalmic disease and that the picture is not distorted by errors of refraction. Major variations in pupillary diameter, and also extreme enlargement or reduction of pupils unaccounted for by light stimulus point to lack of balance in the reactions of the vagus and sympathetic nerves.

Other indications are red or white dermographia, marbled skin, patches of redness in the cheeks or neck region if under mental stress. These patients generally respond very well to 30c and LM potencies. The highest centesimal and decimal potencies should only be given in very small doses.

The third principle therefore is:
— low potencies if vegetative reaction is poor
— medium potencies if vagus and sympathicus are in balance
— high potencies with hyperergic, allergic reactions and vegetative imbalance.

The fourth criterion determining choice of potency considers the patient's vitality and the degree of agreement between patient and drug picture.

Experience has shown that in the final stage of a disease process, reactive potential has become exhausted. A very high potency — perhaps above the 200c — would make demands that go beyond these patients' resources. The precariously maintained regulatory balance breaks down when compelled to respond to such a stimulus. A brief flicker of improvement and the candle goes out, particularly if the drug one has selected fits very well. If on the other hand the patient has considerable vitality and case-taking reveals wide-reaching similarity in mental and constitutional symptoms, it will be perfectly safe to use a very high potency. Good vitality and a good simile will give remarkable cures with very high potencies. Where the drug diagnosis is less certain it is better to make do with medium or low potencies, maintaining observation to see if something better might not come up.

Summary

The choice of potency ranks below the selection of the appropriate drug. For a lasting and 'gentle' cure, it is important to adapt the potency to the case.

The terms 'low', 'medium' and 'high' potency do not refer to absolute values. The standard to be used is the reactivity of the diseased organism. Being a special form of regulatory therapy, homoeopathy calls for individualization in determining both the nature and the power of the stimulus. The toxicology based on material doses and the subtle toxicology of homoeopathic drug tests on healthy subjects show a corresponding affinity of medicinal agents to the level of disorder: organic lesions call for low potencies, functional disorders for medium, and predominantly mental states for high potencies.

The bioavailability of a drug depends on the method of preparation. The pharmaceutical methods used in homoeopathy 'activate medicinal properties that previously lay hidden.' The lowest effective potency for agents which have no medicinal properties in the crude state is at the level of colloidal solubility (about the 8x). Highly toxic materials should not be given in low potencies. In their case, homoeopathic alteration starts only at a level beyond that used in phytotherapy or allopathy — often not below the 12x.

The fact that sick people differ greatly in reactive potential means that the choice of potency has to be adapted to this. A tendency to over-react calls for high and gentle potencies (LM potencies); poor reactors need a 'sledge-hammer'.

High potencies above the 200c should never be given to patients in a parlous state.

The more comprehensive the agreement between disease picture and drug picture, covering also the broad-based constitutional and mental state, the higher the potency selected.

2 Dose

In the examples he gave of drug diagnosis (see p. 124) Hahnemann referred to appropriate potencies and to dose. His first example was that of a robust woman who was given one drop of the mother tincture. The debilitated man whose case has been quoted in this book was given half a drop of the potentized drug.

Potencies up to Loschmidt's number (about the 23x) also relate, at least in theory, to the reduction in the amount of original matter, i.e. the dose. Beyond that point potency is entirely a matter of energies.

These theoretical stipulations must be taken into account when we speak of the dose, i.e. the 'amount' of matter or energy. As no scientific explanation has so far been forthcoming we have to base ourselves on experience and observation.

By the way, in view of all we know to date it is highly unlikely that the problem will be solved with the methods used in materialist science. Modern physics has, however, partly overcome the old concept of matter and may well be expected to produce an explanation of the energetic process of potentization.

Observations made on highly sensitive patients have shown that it is possible to avoid excessive initial aggravation in such subjects by reducing the dose in which high potencies are given.

Example
A schizophrenic patient would show anxiety and restlessness after his weekly 5 drops of *Phosphorus* LM XVIII. When the dose was reduced to one drop he no longer showed this primary reaction. To substantiate this, I gave him 5 drops of placebo on one occasion. The restlessness did not develop in this case.

The opposite may also be the case. Indian colleagues have told me that they get very good results with divided doses. They give high potencies of one particular drug two or three times in succession at 2-6 hour intervals and then allow a long time to pass before repeating the drug.

To my knowledge, the issue of adapted dosage has not been given much consideration so far. There is very little on the subject in the literature. I therefore have to confine myself to personal communications and my own observations.

1st observation: 1 granule of a high potency is sufficient for most infants, debilitated young children and old people in a reduced state of general health.

One drop of a high potency is sufficient for patients with mental conditions, particularly in states of excitement. Manic depressives often need 5-8 drops when in the depressive phase; the closer they are to change-over to the manic phase, the smaller should the dose be.

One tablet of a high potency has the same efficacy as 5-8 drops of the same potency.

2nd observation: Hyperergic patients with enlarged pupils, lively pupillary reactions and excitement coming to expression in their gestures need only small doses — 1 granule or 1 drop.

Hyperergic allergic subjects with narrow pupils and frozen mien react with greatest gentleness to medium quantities of LM potencies, e.g. 5-8 drops perhaps twice daily.

3rd observation. Low potencies (4x-6x) with organotropic affinity may be given in larger doses in acute cases, e.g. 5 drops two or three times for children, 8-10 drops two to three times for adults. In infectious conditions, for pain and in spastic conditions (asthma, pseudocroup a.o.) cumulative dosage in rising potency proves effective (see *Organon* § 248). One starts with a single dose of 5-8-10 drops or 3-5 granules or 1 tablet in a medium potency (the 12x, perhaps, or the 6c). The same amount is then put into half a cup of cold boiled water, left to dissolve, and then vigorously beaten with an egg spoon (not a metal spoon) for 3 minutes, as though whisking egg whites. Having thus potentized the solution by intense mixing, an egg spoon of it is given every 10-20-30 minutes initially and after this at longer intervals, depending on progress; it should be retained in the mouth as long as possible.

4th observation. In chronic cases, treatment with the constitutional drug in rising potency may be helpful (see *Organon* § 246).

Example
Lymphatic child in good general condition with definite *Calc. carb.* symptoms. Prescription: 1 tablet of *Calc. carb.* 6c daily for 6 days; 2-day interval, then 1 tablet of the 7c; 3-day interval, 1 tablet of the 9c; 4-day interval, 1 tablet of the 12c; a week's interval, 1 tablet of the 30c; 10-day interval, 1 tablet of the 100c; 1 month's interval, 1 tablet of the 200c; 6-week interval, 1 tablet of the 1M; 3 or 4 months' interval, 1 tablet of the 10M.

The time intervals may of course be longer or shorter, depending on the reaction, and the course of treatment may also stop at a lower potency. The above is merely a suggestion, not an absolute principle.

3 Repetition of Dose
Let me repeat: homoeopathy is a form of regulatory therapy. Substitution therapy involves medication to make up a deficit. Compensatory therapy has to be continued until the decompensated organ is in equilibrium and can be kept going on maintenance doses. Regulatory therapy on the other hand introduces a stimulus to provoke a reaction. It is senseless to introduce further stimuli whilst the desired reaction is continuing. Homoeopathic medical treatment should therefore be on the following principle:

Give the drug until there is a reaction. Wait and observe the progress of the reaction. Only repeat the drug when the curative process comes to a standstill or becomes retrograde.

Hahnemann's advice in § 246 of the *Organon* is:

Any clearly progressive and obviously increasing amelioration in the course of treatment definitely precludes the repetition of any form of drug treatment whilst it continues. All the good being achieved by the drug the patient has taken is in this case rapidly moving towards completion.

The most important thing if treatment is to be successful is to *watch and wait*. Patience and observation are priceless virtues, though our present age in all its rush knows little of them. We need to learn again that the sowing of the seed and the harvest of the fruit have their seasons. Much is ruined by too much being done too often in our impatience.

There is no fixed rule as to how long one should wait. Every individual, every state of illness, every drug and every potency has its own laws.

The general principle is:

— low decimal potencies may be repeated more frequently
— high centesimal potencies act for weeks or months
— LM potencies are flexible; they may be given daily or we may wait
— if rising potencies are used, the same drug may be given at increasing intervals for an extended period of time.

9

OBSERVATION OF DRUG REACTIONS

Observing the reactions of patients following exhibition of the drug can be almost as thrilling to the homoeopathic practitioner as the solving of a crime.

Before such observations are considered in more general terms, it is important to make critical assessment of the reactions one sees again and again, reactions that are almost inevitable, and differentiate them from the commonly seen placebo 'effects'. The curative effect as such does not furnish ideal proof of efficacy, for placebos will also reduce pain.

It is the specific direction of homoeopathic drug action, with a relatively powerful primary reaction (known as 'initial aggravation') preceding the curative phase, the appearance of side reactions which are in accord with the drug picture, and the fact that recovery follows the standard pattern which differentiate drug action from placebo effect.

The latest fashion in arguments brought forward against all forms of treatment which do not fit the thought forms used in orthodox medicine is to refer to placebo effects. The result cannot be denied — ergo it must be a placebo effect. It is as simple as that! Observe your patients' reactions carefully therefore and distinguish the placebo effects which lack in direction (though we, too, owe a great deal to them) from the regular progress of a specific drug action.

The regular progress of a cure in cases of chronic illness has been formulated by Hering, on the basis of Hahnemann's observations: ideally the curative effect of a drug consists in the mental state improving first of all, after which the physical complaint disappears; in a syndrome shift from above to below (e.g. from arms to feet) or from within to without (internal organs to skin); in the time sequence of pathogenesis running backwards like a film, so that the symptoms which arose last will improve first.

1 Observation of Reactions Encourages a Self-Critical Attitude

Experimental drug tests on healthy human subjects provide the basis for drug therapy. Observation of the patient following exhibition of the drug will demonstrate if the choice of drug, potency and dose in the individual case has been right or wrong. We do not simply accept the statements made by patients without checking them — 'I am better', or 'I have been worse since taking the tablets'. A depressive person suffering from arthritis may say: 'My knee is better, I can walk more easily.' Yet he is as depressed as he was before. Is this kind of reaction all there is? Have we achieved a cure when there is improvement in a symptom? Genuine scientific work begins where we are able to question our own actions. We are able to review our own actions by observing the reactions they produce. This is the essence of scientific work, and we should above all learn from our mistakes.

In my study of the *Organon* I have been particularly impressed by the immense care Hahnemann took over his observations, and the self-criticism he applied in checking the reactions following the exhibition of a drug. After all, it was the childlike naivete and the optimistic belief in the infallibility of their treatments shown by his contemporaries that led him to look deeper. To this day, one often comes across dogmatic 'certainty' being expressed, for instance in applying the findings made in animal experiments all too easily in the treatment of sick humans. One criticism which cannot be levelled at homoeopathy is that drug actions are not conscientiously observed.

2 Initial Aggravation

This is quite common following exhibition of the homoeopathic drug. The term makes us feel uncomfortable, for our aim is to cure and not to make people worse. I would therefore suggest that we use the term 'initial reaction'. Spa physicians use the neutral term 'spa reaction' for the initial aggravation often seen in patients taking the cure. In Hahnemann's view, the cure of a natural illness results from a reaction of the vital energy to the action of the alterative drug. The drug induces the curative process by stimulating vital energy (see § 64 in the *Organon*).

Homoeopathic medication being 'appropriate to the individual case' and in a 'small dose', 'a kind of minor aggravation' arises 'immediately it has been taken . . . in fact, however, it is nothing but a drug-induced illness that is very similar to and slightly more powerful than the original malady' (§ 157 in the *Organon*). 'This minor homoeopathic aggravation' is a good sign in acute conditions (§ 158), for it shows that the choice of drug was correct. If it is too powerful, the potency or the dose was incorrect. Such 'susceptible, highly sensitive patients' (§ 156) are given the drug in its gentlest form when it is repeated, best of all in LM potencies.

Initial reactions should not occur in chronic cases if the correct potency has been chosen, dynamizing further on repetition (see p. 149).

3 Secondary Drug Symptoms

These may appear if the chosen drug does not entirely cover the case and the patient is very susceptible.

Example

A patient presents with a painful inflammation in the basal joint of the thumb. This developed suddenly during the night. The area is red, hot and swollen; movement, jolting and the hand getting cold aggravate the pain. A typical *Belladonna* picture. Prescription: 5 granules of *Belladonna* 200c, a single dose placed dry on the tongue. Presumable clinical diagnosis: gout. Increased serum uric acid levels confirm this the next day. The pain and inflammation disappear within 24 hours. On the third day the patient complains of a humming noise in the right ear, throbbing with his pulse beats, which he notes particularly whilst sitting down. It is markedly better on walking.

Consultation of Hahnemann's *Materia Medica Pura* (vol. 1, symptom no. 340) shows this to be a *Belladonna* symptom. With no further treatment given, the noise disappears in 5 days.

Comment: a) The dose had been too high for a sensitive patient; 1 granule would have been enough. b) *Belladonna* fitted the local condition very well, but not the whole person. The potency was too high, the 30c would have been better. c) The appearance of secondary drug symptoms is a nuisance to the patient but leaves no lasting effect.

A good observer will learn a great deal about the symptomatology in this way and gain experience in the use of the drug. Such incidents confirm the reality of homoeopathic drug tests and the efficacy of high potencies, for such a definitely drug-related symptom would not develop unless there has been something there to cause it. Placebo effects will almost never produce specific symptoms, they will be described in diffuse and indefinite terms. The precisely defined modality 'worse while sitting' and 'better when walking' exactly matches the symptom obtained in drug tests with *Belladonna*.

4 Significance of Symptomatic Aggravation

Symptoms may grow worse at the beginning of treatment or whilst treatment is in progress. This may make both patient and physician lose confidence. The (almost) regular progress of cure must be clearly established in the physician's mind if he is to feel confident himself and also give his patient confidence.

Symptoms getting worse following exhibition of the drug have to be assessed on the basis of location and direction — where they occur and in which direction they shift. A lasting cure proceeds from within outwards. Reversal of this direction is an alarm signal for the discriminating observer. On the other hand we may wait with composure if reactions move in an outward direction: increased mucous secretions, incresed sweats, skin eruptions.

The following are examples of symptomatic aggravation. Assessment would, however, be different in each case.

Reaction following exhibition of drug	*Assessment*
a) 'My knee is more painful, but I am sleeping better.'	Local symptoms getting worse, but patient feels better overall.
b) 'My fear of the future has increased again. Oh yes, walking is better.'	Patient is worse overall, local improvement is of no lasting value.
c) 'My knees are less swollen, but I have a pain in the heart.'	Symptoms moving from periphery to vital organs.

The whole is more important than its parts; the fear a person feels signifies more than their knee; a shift of pathological processes (suppression, metastasis) from periphery to centre may be life-threatening.

The first example shows favourable progress from within outward; the short-term aggravation felt in one part is no cause for concern. The other two reactions make it necessary to take the case again and find out where we have gone wrong. Where have I made a mistake? Did I not get the complete totality of symptoms? Was the sum and essence of symptoms incorrectly determined? Did the patient give an inaccurate or incorrect account of something that is important? Has information been withheld out of ignorance or embarrassment?

The best antidote for untoward reactions in a patient is to find the more appropriate drug. In the third example given above, exhibition of the more appropriate drug elicited the following: 'I think I must be allergic to the new drug; my skin is all inflamed.' Yet there was no spontaneous reference to his heart symptoms; heart sounds were clear, no murmurs. When cautious enquiry was made as to his heart complaint, he almost had to make an effort to remember: 'Oh that — no problem there.'

5 Evaluation of New Symptoms
New symptoms appearing in the course of prolonged treatment for chronic conditions may take three forms:

— Symptoms of the underlying condition which continues to progress
— Symptoms out of the patient's biography
— Symptoms relating to the drug.

Examples

1   A patient was under treatment for recurring processes involving the mucous membranes — now tonsils, now sinuses, now bronchi. Treatment of the local disorder seemed successful on each occasion, with recovery rapid, but the spectrum kept changing. The constitutional drug could not be accurately determined until the patient's mother came for treatment and it proved possible to complete the biographical history. The mother said that she had been too embarrassed to tell her daughter that both she and her husband had contracted tuberculosis 3 years before she was born. They had made a complete recovery. The recurring symptoms therefore did not represent a shift due to treatment, for the tuberculinic taint was the underlying cause. Following exhibition of *Tuberculinum denys* (sudden mucosal reaction, fat, florid) there were no further symptoms.

2   A young man of 22 was very annoyed when a weeping eczema developed whilst he was being successfully treated for chronic recurrent bronchitis (with *Hepar sulph.*). He would not accept my explanation that this was a good sign and that he should soon be completely recovered. His vehemence in dispute, saying that he had never had anything wrong with his skin, confirmed the choice of *Hepar sulph.* I was able to persuade him to let me ring his mother right then and there and in his presence. From 400 km away his mother confirmed that he had had repeated purulent skin inflammations until he was 5. The way she described it this has been a superinfected eczema or recurring impetigo. 'Successful treatment' had finally got rid of it, she said, but after that he had always been coughing during the winter. His mother having explained the situation, it was possible to calm the patient down and feel pleased that treatment was taking us from present to earlier symptoms and from within outwards and therefore in the direction of a cure.

3   A patient with rheumatism provides the last example of treatment going in the right direction, towards a cure, by symptoms moving from above downwards. With a certain irony he said: 'Before treatment started I was unable to take hold of anything with my hands. If we go on like this I'll soon be unable to walk, my feet are that painful.' His rheumatic pain was very much better up above. A new symptom making its appearance was burning pain markedly worse in the metatarso-phalangeal joints and midfoot. Definitely worse in a warm bed. He had been given *Sulphur* in rising potencies. Soon after this, he was able to walk well again.

4   Concerning the third way in which new symptoms may appear I refer readers to the example given of secondary symptoms (p. 153) and to the patient developing lancinating pains in the index finger when treated for too long with *Bromium* (p. 28).

If new symptoms appear it is important to consider if one is not getting a 'homoeopathic drug test' from a sensitive subject. Unlike the serious side effects seen with allopathic drugs, however, such drug symptoms produced by homoeopathic drugs are harmless and will rapidly disappear of their own accord.

6 Direction of Cure. Hering's Law

It was Constantine Hering who formulated the directions of cure referred to in the last section. Feeling much indebted to this great master of homoeopathy, we call them Hering's law.

Hering noted that a certain and lasting recovery from the primary complaint may be expected when the direction in which symptoms are eradicated is:

— **from within outwards**
— **from above down**
— **from the present time to earlier times.**

When these directions are followed we can sit back and wait and predict a successful outcome. On the other hand we must rate it an alarm signal if symptoms disappear in the wrong sequence and above all if the process moves inwards from the periphery. Action will be required in this case. The safest and best antidote is to find the more appropriate drug. This will effect a reversal of direction. All antipsoric drugs have action from within outwards in their pathogenesis — a remarkable contribution made by Hering to Hahnemann's theories on the genesis and cure of chronic diseases.

In his *Lectures on Homoeopathic Philosophy* Kent presented many further observations. A thorough study of this book is well worth while. My present concern has been to demonstrate particularly important reactions shown by patients. Observe your patients to see if the drug action follows Hering's law. If it does there are good prospects of a cure. If it does not, treatment needs to be revised.

10

PARTICULAR DISEASE CATEGORIES AND THEIR TREATMENT

Special investigative techniques have divided medicine into many different specialist fields, yet the 'object' these techniques are meant to serve, the human being, has remained whole and indivisible.

Homoeopathy acknowledges the reality of the whole, indivisible, individual human being by giving a drug chosen on the totality of symptoms.

Local conditions have internal causes (except for injuries inflicted from without).

Skin conditions are not local diseases. They reflect the malady to the outside and should be treated from within rather than suppressed from without.

Hahnemann established important principles for the treatment of mental and emotional disorders. He was one of the first among modern physicians to care for and treat the mentally sick in a humane way. Over 150 years ago he made fairly clear distinction between endogenous and reactive psychoses. Psychosomatic medicine has now become fashionable. It has been the basis of homoeopathic treatment from its inception.

In the treatment of neuroses, homoeopathic medical treatment can enhance the effect of verbal psychotherapy (Ledermann, Schmeer).

1 Anything Particular is Merely Part of the Whole

Julius Caesar wrote of Gaul being divided into three parts. A medical historian would have to say that modern medicine is divided into n parts; it is not possible to give an exact figure, for the process of division is still continuing. New specialists establish themselves, and the special subjects of the past have by now spawned specialists and sub-specialists.

The term 'individual' is only used with reference to healthy persons today. Yet the human being remains indivisible, the way he has always been, even in sickness. It is a comforting thought for homoeopathic physicians and their patients that within this discipline treatment always considers the whole person.

> Genuine treatment applied by a physician to a disorder which has arisen in external parts of the body should therefore be directed to the whole, to the annihilation and cure of the general malady . . ., if it is to be effective, reliable, thorough and helpful. (*Organon* § 190)

It:

> does not need much reflection to see that no . . . external malady can arise, remain where it is and even grow worse . . . unless there are internal causes . . . indeed it is not even possible to think of such a condition arising unless the whole of life has occasioned it, for all parts of the organism are intimately bound up with each other, forming an indivisible whole in our perceptions and functionally. (*Organon* § 189)

2 Local Phenomena

Local phenomena, therefore, should not as a rule be treated specifically. The realization that a particular organ is involved should not narrow drug diagnosis down to a few organotropic drugs. Homoeopathic case-taking endeavours to determine the totality of symptoms, and the choice of drug is based on this:

> With the chosen drug given internally only, the general disease state affecting the body is got rid of together with the local malady and . . . cured together with it, proving that the local malady wholly and entirely depended on an illness affecting the rest of the body and had to be regarded as an inseparable part of the whole, as one of the major and most striking symptoms of the total illness. (*Organon* § 193)

Having thus stated the principle, there remain a few 'local maladies' that do merit the name. External injuries of a part may require medical treatment as well as surgical, orthopaedic and other specialized mechanical measures. Homoeopathy has a number of well-proven drugs to offer which will rapidly deal with the damage caused by physical trauma (see Kent's *Repertory* for 'Injuries' p. 1368; 'Burns' p. 1346; 'Wounds' p. 1422).

3 Skin Conditions

Skin conditions are not 'local maladies.' Yet all the world has always been busying itself with ointments and salves. If there is dry rot in the structure of the house, if there is rising damp, or rain water coming through the ceiling, one surely does not call for a painter and decorator. Instead one gets a roofing expert or a builder to come and deal with the problem. Be that as it may — ointments and paints continue to be applied. Treatment rarely considers the inner causes of a disorder showing on the outside. Yet everybody knows that reeds and rushes grow in wetlands. 'The terrain (the soil) is everything' (Claude Bernard).

The New Testament story of the healing of the lepers makes it quite clear that a cure was not achieved by the external laying-on of hands. Deliverance came from within: Your faith has made you whole. Inner change caused the leprosy to disappear.

Such a change can be initiated by a drug capable of changing the constitutional terrain. Deep-acting constitutional homoeopathic drugs provide the most effective help in skin conditions.

Inside and outside are complementary. As an organ of elimination the skin helps to relieve the burden of a constitutional taint. Once we are fully aware of this function performed by the skin we will no longer act rashly in suppressing such healing diseases. 'Such pernicious external treatment, so widely used to this day, is the most common source of all the innumerable chronic conditions, named and unnamed, that are so much bemoaned by mankind.' (*Organon* § 203)

Outside and inside are complementary. The nature of the skin efflorescence, the appearance of the affected skin, is indicative of the internal disorder and an important symptom within the totality of symptoms. There is no specific for eczema, for warts, for ulcerations, therefore. Many drug pictures have characteristic skin symptoms by which they may be recognized.

Hahnemann has classified the different types of chronic diseases in three groups — scabious conditions, caricous lesions and chancres, terms based on representative skin lesions. His *Chronic Diseases* will be more fully discussed in a later chapter. At this point I merely wish to say the following: *Sulphur* produces a skin eruption associated with marked burning pain and irritation. *Sulphur* is the chief drug for the treatment of the first category, psora. *Thuja* relates to warts, condylomas and benign skin tumours. It is particularly indicated in conditions belonging to the sycotic group. *Mercury* is the principal drug for chronic conditions of the syphilitic type. *Mercury* eruptions may differ greatly in appearance, ranging from dermatitis to suppurating ulcers. Analogous to this, syphilis presents many different forms of skin lesions, particularly in the secondary stage, which has been called the 'ape of dermatology', for it apes every possible lesion.

Dermatology is a science which to this day describes more forms than it explains. This brings it very close to our phenomenological approach where analogies are sought on the basis of presenting pictures. We know from toxicology and clinical use — less so from drug tests on healthy subjects — which morphological skin changes belong to which drug. The appearance of the skin thus is a major symptom in drug diagnosis, one that is reliable. Skin symptoms differ in rank from other pathognomic or local symptoms in drug diagnosis.

The special role played by the skin may well be ascribed to the fact that the skin and nervous system develop from the exoderm during embryological development. The skin has both sensory and neurological functions. Symptoms relating to such functions rank high in the scale of personal valuation.

Summary

1   Do not treat skin conditions externally to suppress them, but treat the internal causes with the appropriate drug. The skin helps to relieve the burden of an internal malady.

2   Most skin conditions are indicative of constitutional taints. Hahnemann discussed this in his *Chronic Diseases*. They point to the nature of the internal disorder.

3   Select the drug on the totality of symptoms, with the appearance of the skin ranking as a major personal symptom. The skin has sensory and neurological functions.

4   It is only in the case of parasitic skin diseases that the skin appearance is also pathognomic. But even then the terrain should not be neglected. The individual skin reaction to parasitic infection points to the appropriate drug. Not everybody gets athlete's foot, yet the organism is ubiquitous.

4 Emotional and Mental Disorders

Getting a cold or a life-threatening infection or becoming an invalid are concepts we find easy to accept. Going out of one's mind, however, becoming a raving lunatic or desperate suicide, a neurotic who destroys himself and his family — these are notions our common sense refuses to accept. Such people are no longer kept in chains in this enlightened age, but they are alien to us. New and magnificent hospitals have been built, their bed-capacity more or less excessive, but little thought has been given to regional mental hospitals in Germany. Is this merely an outward sign? Modern homoeotherapy also fails to pay sufficient attention to this field. Hahnemann and his students often treated patients with mental illness. Evidence of this may be found in the *Organon* and in Jahr's excellent *Allgemeine und spezielle Therapie der Geisteskrankheiten und Seelenstoerungen nach homoeopathischen Grundsaetzen* (General and specific treatment of mental and emotional disorders based on homoeopathic principles) published in 1855.

In Hahnemann's day, the mentally ill suffered great tortures. Instead of healing them, 'these cruel men and women do no more than plague those most pitiable of patients with brutal beatings and other painful tortures (footnote to § 228 in the *Organon*). This is the background to Hahnemann's achievement as a physician when in 1792 he accepted Mr Klockenbring, a violently insane man, for treatment, devoting all his time to him under difficult circumstances, looking after him and treating him as a sick person, with no chains, no padded cell, no electroshock. His psychotropic drugs were herbal extracts. At that time he had not yet developed the method of potentization, nor did he have the data from drug tests — all he had was the will to heal. He approached the sick individual as a physician. Pinel has achieved world fame as the first to advocate a humanitarian medical approach to the mentally ill in 1791. Hahnemann is not mentioned in textbooks of psychiatry. He is unlikely to have known of Pinel's work, for links between France and Germany were tenuous in the tempestuous times of the French Revolution. The question as to who first thought of it is of little importance. Hahnemann was the first to actually do something. He undid the chains and ropes which had been used to 'keep patients under restraint'. 'Tears in his eyes, he would often show me the marks left by the ropes his former guardians had used to keep him in check', Hahnemann said in his reports on Klockenbring.[1]

In §§ 210-230 of his *Organon*, Hahnemann formulated his experience with many mentally ill patients in clear principles. He made careful distinction between endogenous and reactive psychoses, differentiating them from neurotic disorders.

The homoeopathic treatment of psychotic and neurotic conditions calls for a great deal of patience and skill. To avoid homoeopathy losing credibility, only physicians familiar with the diagnostic methods used in psychiatry and also with homoeopathy should make the attempt. Another important requisite is good judgement, so that one does not go beyond the limits of medical treatment, particularly with severe neurotic behavioural disorders. Close collaboration with experienced psychotherapists will often be of greatest benefit to the patient. The limits of psychotherapy can be extended through homoeopathic medicine, and the range of medical treatment by analytical or behavioural therapy.

With the above limits taken into account, Hahnemann's principles can still serve as the basis for homoeopathic treatment in psychoses and neuroses.

To assist communication and present a clear picture, the following is based on the clinical diagnosis and not on the syptomatology. It is known that mixed forms occur and syndromes are not always clearly defined. The nomenclature varies from country to country, and theories and definitions also differ. Kraepelin's terms are no longer generally accepted today.

a) *Endogenous psychoses*: schizophrenias, cyclothymic psychoses. Endogenous refers to anything which is 'cryptogenic' — a modest reference to the fact that *scio ut nesciam* is ancient wisdom. Hahnemann referred to these conditions as physical diseases evolving on the basis of constitutional taints. The mental and emotional symptoms shown by these patients are pathognomic and part of the clinical diagnosis. They are only of secondary importance for the drug diagnosis. The physical symptoms which preceded the mental disorder or are concurrent with it must be determined by taking the biographical history or enquiring of others (family etc.). The physical symptoms define the patient's constitution and therefore the root cause. The mental symptoms are of course part of the totality, yet they only rank second in drug diagnosis.

With psychotic patients, the drug diagnosis is based primarily on constitutional physical symptoms.

Mental symptoms are given first consideration, however, in sudden states of excitement. Hahnemann recommended *Aconitum, Belladonna, Stramonium, Hysoscyamus and Mercury* in these cases (footnote to § 221 of the *Organon*). These drugs are given before or during basic constitutional treatment, depending on the situation, but in alternation, not together.

b) Where the history reveals a definite, logical aetiology to the mental disorder, drug diagnosis will primarily relate to drugs with a similar mental trauma.[3]

Reactive psychoses develop if the constitution cannot cope with powerful mental stresses. The majority of the bereaved overcome most of their pain by working through their bereavement and the wound heals, leaving a scar. Others grow melancholic or rail against their fate. Job bore everything and with sublime humility accepted God's unfathomable will (Kaestner). Not everyone is capable of this. Loss of religious faith is no doubt one of the reasons why mental stress is more apt to lead to mental illness, to neurosis and to addiction in the present day. Once the mental situation has been allayed with aetiological drugs, it will be necessary to treat the constitutional weakness. The totality of symptoms will lead to the appropriate constitutional drug.

c) *Postpartum psychosis* is the prototype of symptomatic psychoses. The repertories list phrases which will help us to find the appropriate drug (page nos. refer to Kent): 'Insanity, puerperal' p. 57; 'Insanity, climacteric period, during' p. 56; 'Insanity drunkards, in' p. 56; 'Mania-a-potu' p. 64. Senile psychosis offers a poor prognosis in the long run. Some delusions and states of confusion may improve for a time (e.g. 'Confusion of mind' p. 13; 'Delusions' p. 20).

Physical symptoms rank highest in the sum and essence of symptoms. Cerebral arteriosclerosis generally is the last link in the chain in the pathogenesis of these disorders. The general paresis of late syphilis is a condition we see only very rarely; my own experience is nil. To exclude it, a serum analysis should be done in any psychotic condition, and not only in older subjects.

5 Psychosomatic Illness

The concept of psychosomatic disease covers a wide area in the literature. The sum and essence of symptoms which forms the basis of drug diagnosis in any kind of illness encompasses the personal totality of physical, emotional and mental symptoms. Hahnemann said that:

> . . . in every case of illness to be treated, the mental state of the patient should be one of the most important symptoms to be included in the sum and essence of symptoms if one wishes to register a true picture of the illness, so that homoeopathic treatment may be successfully applied (*Organon* § 210). This goes so far that in selecting the homoeopathic drug, the emotional state of the patient is often the major determinant, for it indicates the particular individual character . . . (*Organon* § 211). Treatment will therefore never be in accord with nature, i.e. homoeopathic, unless in every case, including those of acute illness, we also consider the symptom of mental and emotional changes. (*Organon* § 213)

Homoeopathy has always based itself on the interrelation of psyche and soma. Hahnemann took it as a matter of course that illness could follow mental alteration. In § 225 of the *Organon* he said:

> On the other hand there are emotional disorders, though these are few in number, which do not base on physical disorder but conversely start from the mind, physical illness being minimal, in consequence of persistent distress, hurt feelings, annoyance, insults and frequent occasions for fear or shock. This type of emotional illness will often, in time, also affect the physical condition, and do so to a considerable degree.

Due to Freud and his successors we now know something about the function of the unconscious, about unconscious errors (errors in writing, errors of speech, mislaying or forgetting things, accidents). Some diseases may be regarded as such errors on the part of the unconscious. They present as physical illness, yet they form a logical part of the biography and have biographical necessity or are a kind of atonement or expiation. V. von Weizsaecker wrote in his *Studien zur Pathogenese* (studies in pathogenesis) that a mental or emotional disorder converting to physical symptoms does not choose the location at random and that there may be a logical connexion between the type of mental disorder and the choice of organ. Practically all homoeopathic drug pictures show correspondences between psyche and specific physical symptoms; both are included in the sum and essence of symptoms and help to determine treatment. In my paper 'A pictorial study of anxiety symptoms',[4] I attempted to show the correlation between the individual form taken by anxiety and fear symptoms and the changes in blood circulation observed in such cases.

The pale, cold anxiety of *Veratrum album* with centralization of the circulation is essentially quite different from the red, hot fear of *Belladonna* where the head is congested, or the congestive, constrictive fear of *Lachesis*. These examples show that with psychosomatic anxiety complexes the particular type of blood distribution — which is always abnormal in such cases — should be included in the sum and essence of symptoms.

Two examples are given below. Paroxysmal tachycardias very commonly are the psychosomatic equivalent of unconscious anxiety states.

Examples

1   Housewife aged 33, mother of three.

Physiognomy: delicate, sensitive type (Huter), very pale, brunette, anxious facial expression, restless gestures, reserved, not much disposed to talk.

Principal complaint: frequent attacks of tachycardia, out-patient and in-patient treatment, brings medical report with her: supraventricular paroxysmal tachycardia. Treatment to date: verapamil hydrochloride, propanolol, digitalized, oxacepam. Eyeball pressure or carotid sinus compression would not stop an attack. ECG between attacks n.a.d.

Spontaneous report: attacks very sudden, no prodromal symptoms. At the same time anxiety and coldness with pain in epigastrium. Arms and legs as though paralyzed, great desire for cold drinks, esp. champagne. Cold sweats, esp. on forehead, 'on the point of collapse, have to sit down or lie down.'

Specific and indirect questions: as a girl, very painful periods, periods at 20-22 day intervals, menses heavy, afterwards completely exhausted. Beyond this, nothing could be elicited.

Husband's report: to save embarrassment I did not question more deeply at the first consultation. The patient's reserve made anything else impossible. The husband reported: attacks more frequent prior to periods; she had been more irritable recently, always restless, would rant at the children, but sexual desire had been increased. Asked why she was so utterly restless, and whether they had talked about this, he said that she prayed a great deal, but this, too, gave her no peace. She felt damned and full of guilt. With some hesitation he told me that the whole thing had started after a miscarriage. In an attack his wife was icy cold, her face looked quite haggard, like someone dead, and her pulse could barely be felt or counted.

Symptoms on which the drug diagnosis could be based: collapse with anxiety and coldness, pallor of face and sweat on forehead. Paradoxically: desire for cold drinks. Anxiety with feeling that she's damned, seemingly religious motives, guilt complex. Pulse rapid and small. Premenstrual aggravation.

Drug chosen: *Veratrum album* LM VI/XIV/XVIII.

Follow-up: frequency and severity of attacks were soon reduced, after 4 months no further attacks. She was more open and approachable. Irritability before menses had gone. Altogether her old cheerful and equanimous self again.

2   Woman aged 54, widowed, with three grown-up children. Husband had been killed in the war.

Physiognomy: nutritional-sentient type (Huter), equivalent to Kretschmer's mixed pyknic/leptosome type; talkative, open, lively gestures and mien.

Principal complaint: had always had rapid heart beats, 'heart beats wildly'. Paroxysmal tachycardia for 10 years.

History: always on medical treatment, verapamil would soon put an end to attacks, but they were always recurring. Many tranquillizers, hormones would improve hot flushes, but very weepy.

Spontaneous report: anxiety states in confined spaces, preferred to use the stairs rather than enter a lift; since menopause hot flushes with sweats, worse in hot, unaired rooms, at night. Great desire to fresh air, kept doors and windows open at home. During an attack she would go out on the balcony — a great help — undo everything (skirt, bra). Did not like tight clothing at all, throat had to be kept cool.

Specific and indirect questions: menopause for 8 years, periods used to be heavy and prolonged, towards the end she would often suffer with headaches, afterwards she felt quite well. Night-time anxiety states, dreams of persecution, she had been through terrible experiences as a refugee at the end of the war. Remembering those days still gave her palpitations. This had nothing to do with her heart attacks, however. Her gynaecologist thought the menopause was responsible.

At the second consultation she told me spontaneously that she had been almost throttled to death during a rape. Since then she felt afraid if anyone even touched her throat. She had struck one of the children on one occasion for grabbing her around the neck from behind; afterwards her heart had been beating very fast for hours.

Symptoms on which the drug diagnosis could be based. Afraid of anything constricting or confined, tightness at throat, desire for coolness and fresh air. Images corresponding to hot, choking fear and the constricting coils of a serpent could also be found in the experiences she had been through, probably triggering the tachycardia via the unconscious.

Drug chosen: *Lachesis* 30c, 100/1000c at long intervals, with sac. lac. inbetween.

Follow-up: the hot flushes were worse for a time but within 3 months had become markedly reduced. Tachycardiac attacks soon became less frequent, returned with greater intensity during the summer and had stopped completely after 1 year. Palpitations still occur if anything comes up suddenly — pleasure, shock, unexpected noises. She continues to feel uncomfortable in hot rooms and in a crowd. It is a real joy to her that her relationship with her eldest daughter has improved so that they are now really able to talk to each other. This one of her children had been old enough to take things in during those terrible months on the run. Had that been a barrier all those years between mother and child?

With psychosomatic conditions, the search for the aetiology in conjunction with physical symptoms often points the way to the central drug which is capable of resolving the conflict. Homoeopathic case-taking undoubtedly has therapeutic value. On the other hand it is wrong to attach too great a value to opportunity given for the patient to give spontaneous utterance to conflict situations. The benefit of this may be considerable, but unfortunately tends to be short-lived unless further work is done to deepen the therapeutic effect in skilfully guided dialogue. The aim in taking a detailed history must always be to explore the mental and emotional state, to help us *understand* the patient. That is the only way of arriving at the totality of symptoms. From this point of view every illness is a psychosomatic process arising from the totality of vital energies out of tune. The origin lies in a sphere where a separation into body and soul is not even thinkable. The living body is what it is because it is ensouled; without the soul it is a dead body. 'It is dead, and being entirely subject now to the forces of the physical outside world it decomposes and is dissolved again into its chemical constituents.' (Footnote to § 10 of the *Organon*)

The current concept of psychosomatic disease covers syndromes where an aetiology can be traced which originated from an emotional experience and manifests in physical symptoms. Hahnemann gave a very accurate description of how disposition (low morbidity) combines with triggering elements from the emotional sphere; this concept is now also to be found in modern textbooks.[5]

Those two factors — disposition and triggering factor — carry different weight in every individual case. The disposition can be seen to form the constitutional background to all chronic diseases. Using drugs relating to the aetiology of mental trauma and following up with constitutional therapy, it is possible to achieve lasting results in many of these cases.

6 Neuroses

The treatment of neuroses should only be undertaken by homoeopathic physicians well versed in the basic principles of the theory and treatment of neuroses. The physician must know his personal limits and the limits of the method he is using. Neurotic disorders which have profoundly affected the core of the personality can usually only be effectively treated in collaboration with a psychotherapist. It is essential to realize that neuroses are fed from two sources. The basic constitution a person is born with, and conflicts in the environment of early childhood (parents, siblings, wider family, social environment) together give rise to neurotic behaviour disorders. An approach limited by ideology to allow only one of these factors will not help the patient.

Neurotic behaviour is partly 'learned', pushed down into the unconscious and suppressed. Psychotherapy aims to 'unlearn' what has been 'learned' and 'suppressed' by making it conscious (Redlich/Freedman). Medical treatment with single homoeopathic drugs may be made part of the process and can greatly enhance the effect of psychotherapy. In many cases where personality structure is still intact homoeopathic treatment combined with psychotherapeutic guidance given to the patient will yield very good results, without recourse to full analysis.

There are certain points to be considered in making the drug diagnosis in such cases. You will recall that drug diagnosis must be in accord with the nature of the disorder, the idea of the particular case of illness (Voisin, Eichelberger) or, as Dorcsi puts it: 'We need to grasp the patient.'

The biographical history provides the basis. The biography will often reveal the aetiology of the presenting symptoms. If a particular mental trauma has set the pattern for neurotic response we are able to use one of drugs relating to mental trauma. This route has proved particularly effective in the treatment of physical symptoms resulting from mental stress, when unresolved conflicts have been displaced and are experienced physically — psychosomatic diseases, traumatic neuroses.

'Traumatic neurosis is the term applied to acute or chronic failure to act the right way resulting from a mental trauma which had caused a previously relatively healthy personality to experience intense fear.' (Redlich/Freedman)

Example

An incident causing fear and shock was found to be the triggering factor in the biography of a stammering child. The choice of drug was determined by the symptom: face as red as a lobster when stammering. *Opium* soon effected a cure.

In the discussion of treatment for psychotic illness, it was said that physical signs and symptoms ranked above pathognomic symptoms of the disease in making the drug diagnosis. A similar situation exists with many autopsychic neuroses. There, too, the disorder has 'finally become remarkably one-sided and almost like a local malady transposed to the subtle, invisible organs of mind and intellect' (*Organon* § 215). If the mechanism of repression produces mainly mental symptoms which are part and parcel of the diagnostic picture of a neurosis, the physical concomitants rank higher for drug diagnosis than pathognomic behaviour. On the other hand mental symptoms rank higher in psychosomatic conditions, traumatic and organ neuroses.

Irrespective of such differentiation between the ranking order of physical and that of mental symptoms with different forms of neurosis it still holds true that remarkable and peculiar symptoms and particularly paradoxical symptoms, as defined in § 153 of the *Organon*, always rank highest, regardless of whether they are physical or mental.

Medical treatment for neuroses will be even more effective in the hands of homoeopathic physicians who have been trained in depth psychology. Paschero was the first, to my knowledge, to point out that the symptoms reported by patients often fail to address the underlying conflict. Drug diagnosis determined by the most obvious symptoms in his view does not go to the core of the neurotic disorder. The most obvious symptoms presenting at the moment tend to reflect secondary processing of the conflict. 'Analysis of the patient's biography provides . . . insight into the true nature of his or her symptoms which lie behind reactive structures or defence mechanisms created by the patient.' 'A homoeopathic physician can only be certain of having prescribed the right drug if he . . . considers the mental symptoms which usually hide behind secondary processing and therefore do not show themselves in the presenting picture; he will then have the complete picture of the disease.[6]

The following case history, which I have slightly abbreviated, demonstrates his method:

A young woman, two children, presented with anxiety, depression, intense headaches, a feeling that she was going out of her mind, fear of death and of being on her own, vertigo, short periods of unconsciousness, menstruation painful and low volume, with amenorrhoea of 1 or 2 months duration, dislike of people, hot flushes to the face, chills and unconquerable jealousy. A year previously, she said, her husband, an officer in the navy, had written home that he had attended a ball. The effect of this had been as though he had been toppled off his pedestal. Since then she had the obsessional idea that her husband was unfaithful, the feeling that she was going out of her mind, and withdrew from other people so that they would not notice her confusion. The lower part of the patient's body was remarkably plump, she had a preference for salty and cold foods, thirst, chronic constipation, tiredness around 10-11 a.m., agitated restlessness with desire to get everything done. Considering the picture in the light of her jealousy which appeared the key symptom, and also taking into account the impression she gave of a shy, sad, embarrassed, passive person, *Pulsatilla* seemed the drug of choice.

The biography revealed that as a child she had been thin and irritable. Divergence — squint — from age 5 to 16 (surgically corrected). Shy, reserved, with sudden paroxysms of weeping. Would not allow her parents to approach in that case, as this increased her despair and she felt an impulse to attack them. This therefore was no passive patient looking for consolation and wanting to be loved — the *Pulsatilla* type — but suppressed enmity towards her parents. Her jealousy was a reactive hatred of her parents.

Following analysis of the biography, the following symptoms were selected: resentment, suppressed enmity, fear of insanity, fear of evil, fear that something might happen to her, refusing consolation from parents, excitement, general tiredness 10-11 a.m., preference for salty foods, obesity of lower half of body.

Repertorization of biographical and presenting symptoms led to *Natrum muriaticum.*

To conclude the history, the following words by Paschero should be very much taken to heart: 'A patient should not be considered the way he presents himself, but the way he really is.'

We know that we must accept the phenomena presented by the patient in an unbiased way. Now it appears we are also asked to interpret those phenomena. This seems contradictory. The problem is resolved if we include the nature of the neurotic disorder with reference to the origin of the conflict as one of the phenomena in the totality of symptoms, and if we relate the patient's biography to the presenting symptomatology.

Because of the particular nature of neurotic disorder, the therapist is forced to look for the root of the conflict. Putting it more simply one might say: The presenting symptoms are merely the product of suppression, an unconscious 'falsification.'

Analogous to this, if someone presents as a deceitful person we seek to get behind the facade, to find out what he wants, who he really is.

With neurotic conditions, drug diagnosis must take into account the nature of the conflict and the particular mechanisms of suppression. The absence of love and affection may trigger enuresis in a child, or a marked tendency to lie, or the need to nibble.

The totality of symptoms includes present and biographical phenomena, the conflict and secondary processing of it. Drug diagnosis must be based on the totality of present and past, that is the only way to achieve a fundamental cure.

These thoughts establish a link with the next chapter which will consider Hahnemann's theory of chronic disease. The acute intermediate stages of chronic illness can only be understood if we recognize the common root, find the totality of symptoms from the biography of the patient, and finally base the drug diagnosis on this.

[1] Quoted from Fritsche [1954].

[2] See Schmeer. Die Homöopathische Behandlung der Neurosen.

[3] See Barthel-Klunker I/12; Dorcsi p. 1-8; Koehler Scriptum 'Psychisches Trauma'.

[4] See Koehler, Eine bildhafte Studie über das Symptom Angst. Engl.: A pictorial study of anxiety symptoms. *Br Hom J* **65**:41.

[5] See Redlich-Freedman, *Theorie und Praxis der Psychiatrie* Bd. 2.

[6] See Paschero. Die homoöopathische Diagnose. The quotes and the case history were taken from this paper. See also: Paschero, Homoopathie als konstitutionelle Medizin — Engl.: Homoeopathy is a constitutional medicine, *Br Hom J* **51**:7.

11

COMMENTS ON HAHNEMANN'S CHRONIC DISEASES, THEIR PECULIAR NATURE AND HOMOEOPATHIC CURE

Medicine as it is generally taught today unfortunately does not concern itself much with the constitution of patients. This is due to the fact that disease is onesidedly seen from the point of view of organic pathology. New endeavours to think in constitutional terms are apparent in all the efforts made towards preventive medicine. In this field, the analysis of risk factors is gaining increasing relevance. It is evident that risk factors are to be found not only in the environment but particularly also in the individual person of the patient, in his inherited and evolving constitution. **Most chronic diseases originate in the patient's constitution.** To deal with them properly we must use drugs which influence the constitutional morbid disposition.

Hahnemann's work *Chronic Diseases* presents a magnificent design for the treatment of constitutional diseases. Some of his theoretical views are based on the state of knowledge in his day and need critical evaluation. It is for ever to his great credit, however, that he tested drugs for the treatment of these diseases and, being an excellent and effective observer, pointed the way to drug diagnosis.

With acute conditions, history-taking can usually be limited to the presenting disorder. With chronic diseases, the history has to encompass the whole biography of the patient, to determine his constitution and morbid disposition.

The ancient physicians and philosophers (Empedocles, Hippocrates, Aristotle) *defined* the different constitutions. Hahnemann on the other hand wanted to *know* why some individuals fall ill over and over again.

Going into the aetiology he found that 'infections' (miasms) may trigger chronic illness, or that this 'tinder of infection' is passed on from generation to generation and responsible for an inborn weakness.

For Hahnemann, chronic disease is 'disease deeply implanted, on the basis of infection or heredity'. He identified three basic forms (psora, sycosis, syphilis) and the drugs relating to them (*Sulphur, Thuja, Mercury* a.o.).

These three basic forms are today seen as a model to describe the trends shown by chronic diseases. These trends emerge if the disease pictures of those infectious states (gonorrhoea, syphilis) are compared with the drug pictures of the related nosodes (*Psorinum, Medorrhinum, Syphilinum, Tuberculinum*) and comparable diatheses (lymphatic, gouty/rheumatic, dyscratic, scrophulous).

A synopsis is given of physical and mental symptoms.

A treatment schedule draws attention to the elimination of inhibiting factors, flanking measures, drug diagnosis and avoidable errors.

National statistics for highly civilized countries show a decrease in acute and an increase in chronic illness. It is indisputably true that modern medicine has reduced the mortality and risks of acute and particularly of infectious diseases. The worrying increase in chronic diseases challenges us to make use of all that homoeopathic medicine has to offer to help these patients.

Hahnemann made many useful suggestions which are of particular significance to us because they were the outcome of self-critical observation. They open up the full and rich potential of homoeopathic therapy.

Observation and critical assessment of his own work made it evident to him that a serious therapeutic problem existed when he did not succeed in achieving full cures in the large group of non-venereal chronic diseases. This serious problem was not due to drugs being insufficiently active; it arose from the method of drug diagnosis. When he first started to treat patients homoeopathically, between about 1790 and 1816, he used drugs selected on the basis of similarity to the presenting symptoms. During that first stage he limited history-taking to a transverse section of the current complaint. This proved very successful in acute diseases. Chronic diseases only responded initially, 'further progress was less favourable, the outcome hopeless.'[1] He judged himself and his method of treatment harshly at that period. Critics should take note of this, for that is not the way of someone given to speculation and ideology. These are the words of a man struggling to find the truth and gain knowledge.

> Thus to discover the reason why all drugs known to homoeopathy do not achieve a genuine cure in the above illnesses, and if possible to gain more accurate and rightful understanding of the true nature of those thousands of chronic illnesses which despite the indisputable validity of the law of homoeopathic cure yet still cannot be cured — has been my most earnest endeavour, occupying my mind day and night since 1816, 1817.[2]

Hahnemann described his observations, research findings and experiments in his *Chronic Diseases*.

First of all he realized that:

> . . . with this type of chronic malady, and indeed in every case of (non-venereal) chronic illness, the homoeopathic physician is not merely dealing with the morbid state presently before his eyes — which he should not consider a morbid process complete in itself nor treat as such. He is in fact dealing with a single aspect of a deep-seated original malady the vast extent of which reveals itself in new bouts of illness coming up from time to time. He therefore should not expect to be able to achieve a lasting cure for those individual morbid conditions on the original premise that they are separate illnesses, complete in themselves, so that they would not recur, nor their place be taken by new and different, even more troublesome symptoms. [He realized] That *consequently he must first of all as far as possible determine the whole extent of all the bouts of illness and symptoms which are part of the unknown original malady*, before he could hope to find one or more drugs which on the basis of their peculiar symptoms show homoeopathic agreement with the whole of the original malady. With these he would then be able to achieve an effective cure and eradication of the state of ill-health in its entirety and consequently also of its individual aspects, i.e. all the fragments of the illness showing themselves in those different morbid conditions. (My italics. G. K.)

The following example harks back to my early days in homoeopathy; it illustrates the two stages in the development of Hahnemann's thought.

The patient was a 3-year-old child.

1st prescription: acute febrile infectious condition. On the basis of similarity with presenting symptoms and signs treated with *Belladonna*.

2nd prescription: 3 weeks later presented with lateral pharyngitis, for which *Phytolacca* 6x was given.

3rd prescription: a month later the mother reported that the child was severely constipated. No urge at all, atonic. *Opium* 30x.

4th prescription: 6 weeks later an impetigo-like skin lesion had appeared on the right cheek: *Viola tricolor* 4x.

5th prescription: 8 weeks later the child presented with inflamed lid margins, kept rubbing his eyes: *Clematis erecta* 6x.

All five prescriptions were 'successful' in that the presenting symptoms improved. The mother accepted this to and fro in the 'shunting yard' as normal. It was what she had been used to with allopathic treatment. Meanwhile I had been studying *Chronic Diseases* and the *Organon* and gained in knowledge. A comprehensive history was therefore taken, to obtain the totality of symptoms. This included a transverse and a longitudinal section, i.e. present and biographical symptoms (see chapter on Case-Taking).

From the biography: milk crust at 2 months, 'taken care of' by applying ointment. Gastrointestinal problems at 4 months, treated in paediatric hospital. Bronchopneumonia at 8 months, treated with penicillin. Recurrent nasopharyngeal infections followed. The presenting general symptoms, the drug type (short, squat, pasty habitus) and the biographical symptoms corresponded to the drug picture of *Calcarea carbonica*. The actions of this drug cover 'all the fragments of the illness showing themselves in the different morbid conditions'.

It is evident from this example that the presenting symptoms only achieve true significance in drug diagnosis if considered in the wider biographical context. In other words: the transverse section of the *existing* state of ill-health provides a number of individual symptoms which must be complemented with comprehensive longitudinal section symptoms indicating the *evolution* of the state of ill-health.

1 Significance of Biographical History

Individual stages of a disease are only part of a whole process. If a fundamental cure is to be achieved, the whole process of the evolution of the disease has to be traced back to its early stages. The totality of symptoms includes the biography. This takes us beyond the apparently well-ordered nosological unity of diagnostic definition of the illness. The five diagnoses made in the case described above were exact definitions of local pathological changes. Treatment proved inadequate because it was limited to individual manifestations of an underlying condition. Biographical analysis makes it clear that individual bouts of ill-health are often only the tips of an iceberg which form a uniform whole beneath the surface of the waves.

This discovery was made for us by Hahnemann: we must get to know 'the original malady in its entirety', the uniform disposition forming the background to the different stages in chronic disease. The individual stages of the diseases are not accidental, unrelated phenomena; they have their ontological origin in the patient as an individual person. If we are able to see this we come to understand the rule which applies to drug diagnosis:

Treat the patient, not his various ills.

Homoeopathy thus claims to treat the individual patient on the basis of his constitution. Here I wish to add the following. If homoeopathy sees the human being as a whole individual, it must also recognize his individual wholeness with regard to his *development* throughout life. His past (history), present (current status) and future (discernible disposition) 'arise from a whole and make a whole' (Paschero).

The biographical history, current status and constitutional signs together form the basis of drug diagnosis in chronic illness.

A fundamental cure can only be achieved with a drug if the drug picture matches the whole of this complex.

2 Constitution and Diathesis

Modern textbooks of medicine or paediatrics discuss individual diseases in great detail but make no reference to such all-inclusive concepts as constitution and diathesis.

Attention given to the constitution and diathesis of our patients is of great practical significance for the whole science of medicine. One often hears the complaint these days that in children liable to infection every individual infection is dealt with by routine antibiotic therapy. The real question as to why these children are prone to recurrent infection is never asked. The pathogen cannot be the real cause; for this has to be looked for in the specific constitution of the individual. Physicians of the past took this to be a matter of course. Are we really as progressive as we like to think we are today?

Concentration on the pathology of organs leaves no room for such concepts in modern medicine, with the inevitable consequence that there also is no therapeutic approach in this direction. The homoeopathic treatment of chronic diseases must go beyond organotropic therapy. Organic lesions are the final stage in the morbid process. As physicians, however, we are obliged to prevent such lesions developing, to control the process so that the final stage is never reached. To achieve this we need a method of drug diagnosis that covers the whole person and his potential development within a lifetime. Every biography has its beginning and a definite sequence of events. The inherited disposition and early environmental influences provide the framework, as it were, for potential development. The weighting of these two factors clearly varies from one individual to another, and between them they give rise to the constitution.

The inherited disposition as such is relatively stable. This has been demonstrated in research on identical twins. On the other hand it can also be moulded and shaped by environmental factors. Psychoanalytical studies have shown it to be particularly amenable to change in early childhood. But factors occurring later in life (mental and physical trauma, infectious illnesses, social environment etc.) can also change the way we react. Disposition and environment interact and interpenetrate throughout life. To my knowledge it was Hahnemann who first pointed out that even the robustest of constitutions may be altered by chronic infections.

'Constitution' is differently defined by different authors. For the purposes of homoeopathic treatment I am basing myself on the definition given by Dorcsi.

Constitution means the inherited *and* acquired physical, emotional and intellectual make-up of a person. It reveals itself in the habit, the basic emotional and intellectual proclivities, and the way the individual reacts to internal and external stress factors.

Dispositions or diatheses develop on the basis of different potentials for illness inherent in the constitution.

Diathesis means the inherited or acquired organic weakness and systemic inferiority which leads to the morbid disposition and specific pathological processes in the evolution of a disease (based on Dorcsi's definition).

THE TEMPERAMENTS IN HUMORAL PATHOLOGY

In accord with the state of the knowledge in their day, the ancient physicians defined the different constitutions and diatheses in terms of basic cosmic elements (Empedocles), humours (Hippocrates) or the quality of the blood (Aristotle). The four Ionic temperaments correspond to those elements, humours and blood qualities.

Empedocles	Hippocrates	Aristotle	Temperaments	Type of Reaction
fire	yellow bile	warm-blooded	choleric	warm and dry
earth	black bile	heavy	melancholic	cold and dry
water	mucilage	cold-blooded	phlegmatic	cold and damp
air	blood	volatile	sanguine	warm and damp

Today we still refer to someone as 'temperamental' in everyday language if they show a certain impulsiveness. In Aristotle's philosophy, 'temperament' was an encompassing term defining the particular nature of a person in body and soul. Flury based his method of homoeopathic drug diagnosis on this comprehensive view of 'temperament'. Dorcsi has developed this further, relating particular drugs to the basic skin type of a patient (warm, cold, dry, moist, red, pale).

HABIT AND TYPE OF REACTION

The ancients established on the basis of careful observation that certain physical types related to the character and morbid disposition of a particular group of individuals. In more recent times, Kretschmer's work attracted attention. This author was able to show, on the basis of ancient knowledge, that in the field of psychopathology slender leptosome types are predestined to show schizoid reactions, robust athletic types epileptoid reactions and pyknics cycloid reactions.

Lampert and Curry determined the different types of reaction in the autonomic system relating to different physical types. Carl Huter has given clear directions in his psychophysiognomy as to how the mental and emotional state of a person and his morbid disposition may be established by considering habitus, mien, gestures and speech. He has expanded the older concept of physiognomy.

BIOGRAPHY AND CONSTITUTION
The biography of a patient surveys the processes which have run their course, the past of that person, the evolution of the morbid process. Biographical data usually follow a particular sequence. Case-taking marks the point where the patient's past and future meet. We record the biographical data, relate them to the strange and peculiar symptoms presenting at this moment (*Organon* § 153), and determine the constitutional background on the basis of typology (objectively observable data relating to physique, gestures, mien, speech). Once the constitution has been established it is possible to assess organic weaknesses and systemic inferiority (Dorcsi), i.e. the diathesis. Biography, personal symptomatology and objective signs do not come together at random; there is an underlying order to them which is based on the constitution of the individual. When we recognize the constitution we have the ordering principle governing past, present and future. This order arises out of the totality of an indivisible life; it points the way to the whole. Triggering moment (aetiology), modalities, localizations and sensations belonging to the morbid process have their real basis (Flury) in the constitution, and this comes to expression in physique, in a person's mental and emotional responses and in his or her temperament. Hahnemann did not himself define that real basis to chronic diseases; we are, however, indebted to him for something of even greater significance.

3 Aetiology of Chronic Diseases
Hahnemann found and tested the drugs which make it possible to treat constitutional weaknesses and therefore diatheses.

To find the appropriate drug he started with the history and observation of the patient.

The question to be asked is 'What observations may be made on the history of chronic patients who do not recover fully following exhibition of a well-selected homoeopathic drug? Hahnemann traced the course of the disease back to its aetiology, to the point where the history indicated that something of import had occurred. He noted that the triggering factors in chronic illness might differ quite considerably.

a) Long-term *drug abuse* resulting from exhibition of 'powerful, heroic drugs in large and increasing doses' (*Organon* § 74).

b) Exposure to harmful but avoidable factors: consumption of harmful food and drink; excesses that undermine health; nutritional deficiencies; unhealthy housing conditions, lack of exercise, physical and mental overwork, living in constant vexation (see *Organon* § 77).

c) Looking at the past history of his chronic patients, Hahnemann found that specific skin changes had in many cases appeared at some time prior to the onset of chronic disease of many years duration. He found three types of skin changes merited particular attention:

— Irritating skin eruptions causing the patient to scratch.

— Pointed or cockscomb-like condylomas in the urogenital region.

— Sores in the genital region with inguinal glands hard and swollen.

He knew that condylomas were connected with gonorrhoea and the sores (chancres) with syphilis, both of them contagious diseases. Pathogenic organisms had not yet been clearly defined in his day and he therefore used the term generally applied to contagious agents in his day — miasm.

MIASMS

The term does not usually mean anything to modern physicians, as the history of medicine receives scant attention nowadays. (This is regrettable, for among other things a study of the history of medicine would soon cure us of the arrogant assumption that medicine really only came into its own in the twentieth century and that the healers, priest physicians and physicians of earlier times were ridiculous fools.)

The Greek *miasma* literally means 'pollution.' From Hippocrates's day the term was used to describe morbific agents in the atmosphere, 'exhalations' from the soil causing epidemics. The communicable nature of epidemic diseases was known in pre-bacterial times, the organisms were not.

> Genuine natural chronic diseases have come about through a chronic miasm. Left to themselves and without drug therapy directed specifically against them, they continue to increase, getting worse even if mental and physical dietary regimes are at their best, with the sufferings the individual undergoes increasing all the time, to the end of his life. Apart from those due to medical mismanagement these are the commonest and most serious tormentors of the human race, for the robustest of constitutions, the best regulated mode of life and most active of vital energies are unable to eradicate them. In conjunction with a mode of life beneficial to body,

soul and spirit, they often go unrecognized for several years in young men during the best years of their youth and in girls whose menstrual cycles are regular in the early stages; those affected appear perfectly healthy to friends and relatives, as though the illness which *through infection or heredity*[3] has profoundly marked them had completely vanished; in later years, however, it will inevitably reappear when untoward events or conditions pertain in life. It will then increase all the faster and be much more severe in character the more the vital principle has been put in disarray by destructive passions, grief and worry, and above all by inappropriate medical treatment. (*Organon* § 78, with footnote)

We are aware of the significance of the first two aetiological factors (drug abuse, harmful elements that are avoidable) and how to deal with them. Inevitably we have to exercise our medical and educational functions again and again because of them. The third aetiological factor, the chronic miasm, is, in Hahnemann's terms, **'illness profoundly marking them through infection or heredity'.**

Here again Hahnemann was ahead of his time. He pointed out, for instance, that 'minute but murderous living entities' caused the infection in cholera. He suspected that there must be specific pathogens for different epidemics and — this is the crucial point — that some of those pathogens were involved in the aetiology of chronic diseases. It is not surprising that his ideas would meet with rejection from his contemporaries. Not only did his opponents wax triumphant as such 'nonsense', but many of his students also broke away.

Today we take it as a matter of course that micro-organisms play a role in the triggering of chronic disease. We are familiar with spirochaetes, with the tubercle bacillus, and the viral origin of a number of malignant conditions is under discussion. We know that focal toxic processes can trigger auto-immune disease or chronic rheumatic disease.

Recent discoveries concerning slow virus infections show that Hahnemann's intuitive concepts can be scientifically demonstrated to to be true 150 years later: **Many chronic diseases are originally due to infection.**

INHERITED DISPOSITION
We also know the other half of his statement to be true: 'illnesses profoundly marking them through infection or *heredity*'. Inherited disposition and infection are the 'real basis' on which chronic diseases develop.

The constitutional element is given too much prominence today in discussing the problems of chronic diseases. To my view, the special merit of Hahnemann's theory of miasms is that it presents the possibility of curing the *consequences* of chronic infections which *alter* the constitution.

It is of course important not to take Hahnemann's concept of miasm too far and call everything that causes illness 'miasm'. Unclear definition leads to confusion. Conflicts in early childhood constituting the mental trauma which has significance in psychoanalytical theory (Freud) and for homoeopathic drug diagnosis, should not be confused with miasm.

INTERPLAY BETWEEN INFECTION AND CONSTITUTION

Experience has clearly shown that constitutional disposition is a key element in chronic infection. Not every person exposed to the tubercle bacillus contracts tuberculosis. There is interplay between constitutional disposition and the pathogen's ability to prevail. Every infection produces an engram in the reticuloendothelial system, in the immune mechanism, and consequently alters our inherited constitution. When blood titres of some infectious agent or other are tested one finds that the level of contamination among the population is surprisingly high. Chronic miasms are a reality and can be demonstrated as such. When we take a patient's history, the question as to since when he or she has had the illness, or what happened originally, will often elicit this type of reply: 'he's been coughing ever since he had the measles'; 'she's had asthma since she had whooping cough'; 'the eczema came up after vaccination'. An allopath will hardly know what to do with such information. We are able to give the appropriate nosode or select the drug appropriate to the original infection.

Nosode therapy was developed by Hahnemann's successors, though it follows from miasm theory. If the constitutional factor only is considered, we miss an opportunity of achieving a cure by means of specific nosode therapy; auto-immune therapy with the patient's own blood in homoeopathic potency (Imhaeuser);[4] elimination of toxic foci; influencing symbiosis in the intestinal flora, and other methods.

Both elements — *intra vitam* infection and constitutional weakness — have to be taken into account in deciding on treatment. Homoeopathic drug diagnosis bases on the symptoms given in the history and the observable signs in the individual case. We thus record the morbid phenomena arising from 'infection or heredity'.

Following this general review let us return to Hahnemann's theory of miasms. Below, a summing-up is given of the essential points relating to effective treatment, i.e. to drug diagnosis.

4 Acute and Chronic Miasms

Hahnemann distinguished between acute and chronic miasms. His acute miasms included those causing smallpox, measles, whooping cough, scarlet fever, mumps, the plague, yellow fever, cholera and the different 'fevers which affect many people in epidemics, from a similar cause and with very similar symptoms . . . showing specific characteristics on each occasion' (*Organon* § 73). These are the influenza epidemics due to different virus strains as we know them today, different Salmonella infections, etc.

The essential difference between acute and chronic miasms is in Hahnemann's view that either the vital energies of the patient are able to overcome the acute miasm of their own accord or else the miasm rapidly overcomes the vital energies. Recovery or death are the outcome of acute miasmatic disease.

Chronic miasms on the other hand:

> show . . . such persistence and endurance that . . . they continue to increase over the years, and for the rest of the patient's life cannot be ameliorated, let alone overcome and eradicated, by the inherent powers, however robust his constitution, even if the mode of life and diet are as healthy as they may be, growing worse until he dies.[5]

Only medical (homoeopathic) treatment can overcome them.

The difference between acute and chronic diseases lies not so much in the time they take; the essential difference is whether the organism is able to overcome the illness by itself or medical treatment is necessary to achieve this end.

A third characteristic of chronic diseases is that they occur in phases with latent periods in-between, appear to have been cured but recur 'year after year, having undergone a greater or lesser degree of change and furnished with new symptoms, becoming increasingly more troublesome.'[6]

Hahnemann's final observation is that these miasmatic chronic diseases proceed from the outside to the inside. The first changes occur in the skin. The condition then gradually progresses from the skin to the mucous membranes and vital organs. Skin and mucosal symptoms serve to relieve the internal problem. For as long as the skin efflorescence is maintained, 'the disease as a whole is most easily cured with specific drugs given internally'.[7]

If the relief function of skin and mucosa is suppressed (external applications, surgical intervention, cauterization), the internal process will inevitably spread much more rapidly and grow more and more severe (see chapter on Skin Diseases). The conclusion to be drawn from this is an important therapeutic principle:

Avoid any form of suppressive external treatment. Many chronic conditions are the result of suppression.

Table 9: Differences between Acute and Chronic Miasms

	Acute	*Chronic*
Prototype	measles	syphilis
Duration	brief	life-long
Spontaneous recovery	possible	not possible
Progress	uniform	in phases (primary, secondary, tertiary syphilis)
Direction	from inside to outside prodromal symptoms followed by exanthema	from outside to inside ulceration followed by tabes dorsalis

Syphilis, a condition presenting in many different forms, was taken as the basic example of chronic miasmatic disease by Hahnemann. The clear evidence of unicausal genesis must have held great fascination for him: one single miasm producing so many different stages of the disease that all the individual branches would appear to be individual diseases unless the root cause was known. Hahnemann was one of the first to realize that chancres, the primary lesions of syphilis, must not be treated surgically or with 'caustic, burning or drying agents' as this will cause the disease to progress all the more rapidly. He also called syphilis 'chancriform disease', referring to the primary lesion. His drug of choice was *Mercurius solubilis.*

The second type of miasmatic disease is 'condylomatous disease' or 'sycosis.' This relates to gonorrhoea. Hahnemann already differentiated it clearly from nonspecific urethritis.[8]

The local skin lesions, the condylomas, are acuminate warts which may be cauliflower- or cockscomb-like. They are merely considered a secondary symptom of gonorrhoea today, but we may as well continue to use the term 'sycosis.' Hahnemann also included rheumatic conditions under this heading. Gonococcal arthritis and gonococcal serosynovitis were quite common remote systemic complications in his day. Systemic complications of gonorrhoea have become so rare nowadays that the younger medical generation are not aware of them, probably due to successful early antibiotic therapy. I recall seeing postgonorrhoeic skin eruptions and septic conditions in the skin clinic in my student days. I am mentioning this here because in my experience younger colleagues tend to consider gonorrhoea a minor local problem. The most important drugs for the treatment of sycosis are *Thuja, Natrum sulph.* and in later stages *Acidum nitricum.*

Hahnemann added a third chronic miasmatic disease to syphilis and sycosis, 'the condition which may be given the general name psora (internal form of itch, with or without skin eruption).'[9] 'Just as protracted as syphilis and sycosis and therefore also not becoming extinct, unless radically cured, before the last breath is taken in even the longest of lives . . . the itch (psora) over and above this is the oldest and most hydra-headed of all chronic miasmatic diseases.'[10]

This group of diseases owes its name to the irritating skin changes that are the first manifestation, causing the patient to scratch. The question as to how to define psora or the itch is one that has to be faced in an age when we are accustomed to pinning down the pathogen in every detail. In the case of syphilis and sycosis the organisms are known; with psora we are in the dark. Medical historians have shown that Hahnemann was familiar with scabies. Yet if he had thought the itch mite responsible for psora then surely he would have mentioned this. At an earlier date he had recommended washing with sulphureous water as a sensible treatment for scabies.

Psora goes far beyond this, however, and we do not do justice to Hahnemann's concept of chronic diseases if we define it as the sequel of scabies. In Hahnemann's view, 70% of chronic diseases are of the psora type. Furthermore, a psoric taint is the precursor and cause of the other types of chronic disease. In view of the large number of drugs he listed as suitable for the treatment of psora we may justifiably say that psora is not unicausal, i.e. not due to a single pathogen.

Explanations and theories are true or false for a limited period only. Irrespective of whether the different interpretations of psora are right or wrong the fact remains that to this day the drugs Hahnemann recommended for this type of disease still prove effective. Many brilliant minds have stated and will go on stating that the theory of miasms is wrong, but all those papers and disputes have not cured a single patient. I refuse to take part in the heated discussion of a theory which may be right or may be wrong. My intention is merely to show the way in which chronic diseases can be cured and indicate the points to be considered in making the correct drug diagnosis. In this respect,

Hahnemann has given invaluable advice, and it is up to us to relate his working hypothesis to the present state of knowledge.

The old concept of constitutions had its basis in humoral pathology. This also indicated the direction treatment would take: the humours had to be brought into balance again. The radical purges and derivative treatments to which Hahnemann objected so strongly were the last, badly distorted echo of that old philosophy. Like every end stage in human history, that epoch was merely an exaggerated caricature of what had previously been an effective and meaningful form of treatment.

Hahnemann was a progressive. He had intuitive perception of the era of bacteria and viruses which was to come, taking it into account in his system of treatment. He linked the old theory of constitution with the new concept coming in: chronic diseases have their origin in 'infection or heredity'. Observation and intuitive perception of his chronic patients led him to distinguish three groups of diseases, each with characteristic initial skin changes. He related three diseases and their causal agents (miasms) to those three groups. It was not enough for him, however, to have established a system; he found and tested the drugs which will cure those diseases. It is those drugs which are of primary interest; the system merely provides a retrospective explanation. (NB: The last statement represents my personal view which I have no wish to impose on others. Comparison with the life work of other men of genius throws light on what may appear a paradox: knowledge of 'how to get there', finding a solution, often precedes the search for substantiation. Discovery comes first, theoretical proof follows later.)[11]

The drug pictures of the drugs Hahnemann suggested for the treatment of these disease categories include many phenomena relating to the associated infections. On the other hand they cover many more symptoms and are more comprehensive.

The disease pictures of syphilis and gonorrhoea thus provide the models for similar disease processes. They are not identical with them. Bacteriology and Virchow's cellular pathology have set different standards than those pertaining in Hahnemann's day.

The three types of chronic disease cannot be considered nosological, pathogenetically defined entities with their pathogens accurately definable. They are not in the same category as clinical syndromes with exactly defined pathological anatomy and pathology.

Hahnemann described the different modes of reaction seen in chronically ill patients, modes of reaction which may be due to suppressed or inadequately treated infections or to hereditary causes. Many of the symptoms relating to the different modes of reaction resemble those arising from sequelae of syphilis or gonorrhoea.

Anyone finding it difficult to accept such similarity of symptoms should remember that modern medical nomenclature often refers to similar features with similar names: epileptoid or epileptiform, schizoid, psoriatiform, rheumatic types of illness, atopy, allergosis.

It is interesting to note that the 'actual' disease and processes similar to it often respond to the same treatment. Modern medicine puts much emphasis on specificity; yet the same drug will influence many different reactions in the diseased organism, the number of potential reactions available to the organism being limited.

There is therefore no point in insisting on unicausal origins for Hahnemann's chronic diseases, though in his day they were a fair assumption. Description of the disease process leads directly to therapy; it is the drug that matters. We may know the causal origin or we may not; what matters is that we know which drug will achieve a cure.

The first and most important drug in the treatment of psora is *Sulphur*. Homoeopathic drug tests with *Sulphur* showed the skin to be the primary target; it turns rough, with poor healing tendencies and an inclination towards eczematous changes, infected pustules and boils. Severe irritation causes the person to scratch and the irritation then becomes a burning sensation; everything worse in a warm bed and on contact with water. Irritating skin affections causing the patient to scratch are the first characteristic sign of psora, hence the name 'the itch'. Suppression of the relieving skin manifestations leads to involvement of the mucosa and internal organs. The total drug picture of *Sulphur* makes it clear that practically every organ and tissue may be involved. The interaction which exists between skin, mucosa and internal organs gives an idea of how psora develops and how *Sulphur* can be effective in the treatment of psoric disorders. Treatment with the drug may cause suppressed skin and mucosal processes to recur for a time. Successful treatment first cures the internal disorder and then the skin (see Hering's Law).

August Bier has shown that:

... exhibition of elementary *Sulphur* caused a high degree of mobilization of tissue sulphur which was then eliminated. How may this be interpreted? I assume the people concerned had extreme cumulation of sulphur in the organism, that their sulphur metabolism had become abnormal and that the small dose of elementary *Sulphur* provided a stimulus for the elimination of excess sulphur.[12]

Psoric drugs above all include the major elements found in the body and trace elements with katalytic function [homoeopathic drug names in italics, added in parentheses where terms differ — translator]: calcium (*Calcarea*), potassium (*Kalium*), sodium (*Natrum*), *Magnesium*, silica (*Silicea*), *Phosphorus*, nitrogen (compounds), *Sulphur*, carbon (*Carbo*), their compounds and acids, pure clay (*Alumina*), antimony (*Antimonium crudum*), arsenic (*Arsenicum album*), *Barium*, copper (*Cuprum*), tin (*Stannum*) and zinc (*Zincum*). Particular plant drugs mentioned by Hahnemann were *Lycopodium*, *Mezereum* and *Sarsaparilla*. His followers have made changes and additions to the list. Any drug with a sufficiently wide spectrum of action may prove the similimum in an individual case. **The law of similars ranks above the merely theoretical psora concept.** Psoric drugs are never prescribed on the suspicion that there may be psora, but only if the totality of symptoms for a psoric patient matches the drug picture of the psoric drug in question.

The fact that the major psoric drugs are important building stones in the body or elements with katalytic function points the way to a rational explanation of psoric disorders. August Bier's work on sulphur metabolism has shown that potentized *Sulphur* can effect the elimination of excess sulphur via the gut and skin. Analogous to this it may be argued that potentized elements may well be able to correct metabolic disorders relating to them. We are indebted to Bier and Mezger for work done in this field.

> Analogous to this the obvious conclusion would be that other minerals, apart from sulphur, are also present in the wrong proportions in the organism and may give rise to disorders of mineral metabolism which it may be possible to correct by giving the mineral in question in small doses. This could also mean that there is rhyme and reason to the way homoeopathic physicians insist, apparently against all reason, that common salt, which we ingest in large quantities day after day, is a highly effective drug if given in homoeopathic preparation and dosage. There is plenty of evidence that sodium chloride metabolism is frequently out of order.[13]

Mezger was able to produce similar evidence for *Magnesium carbonicum*.[14] To avoid misconception let it be clearly stated however that we are not dealing with substitution therapy in this case but the use of potentized drugs to regulate a primary functional imbalance.

Example
A boy aged 18 months presented with rickets and occipital sweats; craniotabes despite exhibition of cholecalciferol and calcium preparations. Prescription: *Calcarea carbonica* 12x b.d.

Two weeks later no more head sweats; 8 weeks later no acute signs of rickets. There had been no changes in life style and diet during this period.

Voegeli called psora a 'constitutional disorder in the assimilation of essential minerals in the body'.[15] In the example given above it must be assumed that the child had a congenital weakness relating to calcium utilization. Substitution would have no effect in such a case.

Mezger noted that:

> . . . the *Magnesium* constitution tends to run in families. It is important to take note of this when *Magnesium* has proved highly effective in a patient. One will often find other cases among the blood relations who may have presented us with quite a headache before but will be found to respond very well to *Magnesium*. Having made many observations of this kind I consider the hereditary nature of the *Magnesium* constitution . . . to be definitely established'.[16]

Cellular deficiency due to abnormal utilization of an essential element gives rise to specific symptoms characteristic of that particular element. This is why there is not just one drug for the treatment of psora. It is necessary to make a very careful study of the totality of symptoms in order to establish the particular disorder in the individual case.

Drug diagnosis can be difficult if two or three such disorders are concurrent. In most of these cases a compound drug emerges and we may establish the symptomatology of *Hepar sulphuricum* (*Calcarea* and *Sulphur* symptoms side by side), for instance, or of *Calcarea silicata*, *Calcarea phosphorica*, etc.

5 The Drug Pictures of Chronic Nosodes

Four different approaches may be used to gain a clear understanding of the nature of the three types of chronic disease:

a)   Comparison with the disease pictures of the infectious diseases serving as models and with those of disorders of mineral metabolism
b)   Knowledge of the drug pictures of the related nosodes
c)   A study of the relevant diatheses
d)   A study of the drug pictures of the principal psora drugs given by Hahnemann.

In my view, a thorough knowledge of the drug pictures of the related nosodes is particularly important.[17]

Type of disease	*Nosode*
Psora	*Psorinum*
Sycosis	*Medorrhinum*
Syphilis	*Lueticum* (*Syphilinum*)

It is known that Hahnemann did not think much of the nosodes, isopathy being suspect to him (see footnote to § 56 in the *Organon*).

Hahnemann accepted nosodes deriving from similar diseases in animals, but he warned against the use of nosodes deriving from the morbid products of the same human disease the patient is suffering from. Present-day experience bears this out. A fresh tuberculosis may be aggravated on exhibition of *Tuberculinum Koch exotoxin (Tuberculinum residual)* (Koch found this out, but he had not read the *Organon* of course). *Psorinum* will not cure scabies but it will be effective in the treatment of eczematous changes that are similar in appearance and cause skin irritation 'as if' itch mites were burrowing.

The drug picture of *Psorinum* is multifaceted. A number of psoriatic drugs may be discerned within it, for it has the unpleasant body odour and the skin eruptions of *Sulphur*, the debility of *Phosphorus*, the sensitivity to cold of *Calcarea*, *Kalium*, *Magnesium* and *Silicea*, the lack of self-esteem shown by *Silicea* and *Calc. carb.*; ravenous appetite during the night reminds of *Phosphorus*, the persistent constipation of *Calc. carb.*, enlarged lymph glands of *Calc. carb.*, *Baryta carb.* and *Magnesium carb.*

Table 10: Most Commonly Used Drugs

Psora	*Sycosis*	*Syphilis*	*Tuberculinic*
Principal elements in the organism:			
Calcarea	Thuja	Mercury	Phosphorus
Kalium	Natrum sulph.	Acid.nit.	Stannum
Natrum	Acid.nit.	Aurum	
Magnesium		Iodum	
Phosphorus		Kalium bichr.	
Silicea		Kalium iod.	
Sulphur		Plumbum	
their compounds		Thallium	
and acids			
Trace elements:			
Alumina			
Antimonium crudum			
Arsenicum album			
Barium			
Cuprum			
Zincum			
Plant drugs:			
Lycopodium			
Mezereum			
Sarsaparilla			
Nosode:	Nosode:	Nosode:	Nosode:
Psorinum	Medorrhinum	Syphilinum	all the Tuberculinum nosodes

PSORINUM

Source: Secretion from scabietic vesicle.

Drug test: Hering, 1834, with the 30x potency.

General aspects: 'Offensive to sight and smell is the subject who needs this medicine' (Kent). Debilitated, emaciated, chilly — warmly dressed even in summer. Paradoxically also profuse offensive sweats.

Principal action: Functional and psychosomatic disorders, fear, hypotension, skin, mucosa, lymphatic organs, allergies.

Mentals: Lack of self-esteem, inferiority complexes, nervous, fear of the future, all is dark around him. Hopelessness, despair, Misanthrope, psychasthenic, neurasthenic. Poor memory.

Nervous system: Attacks of migraine, occipital or frontal headache improved from eating, better if head warm, better following nosebleed; worse from cold draughts, suppression of skin eruptions or of menses.

Skin: Looks unwashed and uncared-for (*Sulphur*). Dry or greasy. Seborrhoea sicca or oleosa. Skin eruptions with pustules, papules or vesicles, weeping. Scabs. Marked skin irritation, worse in warm bed and from washing.

CVS: Hypotension.

Gastrointestinal: Hunger at unusual times, gets up during the night to eat something. Stools: mostly atonic constipation interrupted by offensive diarrhoea. Offensive flatus smelling of rotten eggs.

Respiratory organs: Chronic coryza, blocked nose, retronasal discharge. Frequent sore throats, tonsils hypertrophic. Marked lymphatic reactions. Allergies: hayfever, sometimes with asthma, alternating with eczema. Cough worse in winter, in cold air. Dyspnoea, restrosternal pressure.

Modalities: Worse in winter; in cold air; before a thunderstorm; from pressure; when walking, sitting, standing; following suppression of physiological eliminations or skin eruptions. Better from warmth, food, lying down.

Summary

Debilitated, emaciated, chilly subjects with offensive sweats; appear unwashed and uncared-for.

Anxiety and inferiority complexes: Functional and psychosomatic disorders; allergies.

Skin, mucosa and lymphatic system predominantly involved. Alternation of dermal and mucosal processes; alternation between eczema and asthma. Hypotensive and hypotrophic.

MEDORRHINUM

Source: Gonorrhoeal urethral secretion.

Drug test: Swan, 1880.

General aspects: Often indicated with sequelae of inadequately treated gonorrhoea, vaccination, serum injections, foreign protein.

Principal actions: Inflammatory conditions in urogenital region. Gouty or rheumatic conditions. Proliferative changes in skin and mucosa, benign growths such as warts, condylomas, polyps, cysts. Neurotic syndromes, hallucinations. Depression with thoughts of suicide.

Mentals: Irritable, in a hurry, restless, time passes too slowly. Despairing sadness with thoughts of suicide; often highly changeable state of mind — sad, morose and hasty in the mornings, more relaxed in the evenings and during the night. Weeps when talking of his illnesses, sensible of his sufferings just from speaking of them (like *Acidum oxalicum*).

Sensitive, has premonitions, tends to predict disaster. Hallucinations: hears voices; others talking about him; someone standing behind him. Poor memory; forgetful; short-term memory particularly bad. Forgets what he was about to do; forgets names of people he knows well. Poor spelling, makes spelling errors because of inner haste and lack of attention. Starts many things, but does not finish. Unsystematic, confused, no definite goal. Jumps from one idea to another when talking.

Nervous system: Headache with sensation of band across forehead. Pain in occiput going down to nape and spine. Neuralgia comes and goes suddenly, worse in cold damp weather, better from rubbing and movement. Left-sided sciatic pain with dirty coated tongue and feeling of acidity in stomach.

Secretions: Elimination of toxins through mucosa — acrid offensive discharges, smelling of fish brine. Thick, jelly-like.

Respiratory organs: Nasal secretion viscid, white or yellowy. Nose blocked, tip of nose often cold; itching and biting in tip of nose. Tonsils enlarged. Adenoidal hypertrophy, prone to infection. Cough: dry and painful, worse at night and in warm room, better when lying prone. Asthma: better in knee-elbow position, by the seaside (except in cold, dry weather). Attacks worse during the day, during thunderstorms.

Digestive organs: Marked thirst. Often ravenous, even immediately after a meal. Desires stimulants such as alcohol, tobacco, sweets, salt; often also green fruit, sour things, ice. Foul breath in the mornings. Cramp-like pain in solar plexus with extreme oppression, worse from thinking of it and better lying prone. Chronic constipation with sticky, clayey stools; often only able to pass stools if leaning backwards. Perianal and gluteal erythema of infants.

Urogenital system: Pelvic region is particularly affected in the *Medorrhinum* picture, with inflammation of the bladder, kidneys, prostate, ovaries, adnexa, uterus. Urine has offensive smell of ammonia.

Greenish fluor, smelling of fish brine, with marked irritation of external genitalia. Menses heavy, with offensive smell, at the same time breasts are sensitive and painful. Libido increased after menses. Breasts icy cold, particularly around nipples, marbled skin.

Locomotor system: Acute and chronic rheumatic complaints, worse in wet cold weather, better by the seaside. Deformed finger joints. Pain in heels and soles of feet, with cold sweats, in shoulder and sacral region; hip joints, radiating to thighs.

Skin: Cold, damp, stinking sweats. Cold skin in extremities, nose, breast. Proliferations in skin and mucosa — warts, acuminate and pedunculate, acuminate condylomas, polyps. Brittle nails, deformed nails with transverse grooves. Yellow spots on dorsum of hands. Erythema on buttocks and perianally in infants.

Modalities: Worse during the day if thinking of the complaint; cold, touch, inland, by inland waters and in damp river valleys. Better late evening and at night (above all mentally); prone or knee-elbow position; firm rubbing; by the seaside.

Summary

Irritable, hurried, restless subjects who find the time passes too slowly. Alternation between morning depression and relaxed mood in the evening.

Neurotic disorders with distrust of self and others; short-term memory poor. Hallucinations. Poor spelling.

Lacks system, confused, no definite goal. Depression with thoughts of suicide.

Inflammatory conditions in urogenital region; gouty and rheumatic complaints. Proliferations in skin and mucosa (warts, condylomas, polyps, cysts). Many symptoms worse during the day and from damp cold climate.

SYPHILINUM (LUETICUM)

Source: Secretion from syphilitic chancre.

Drug test: Swan, 1880.

Principal actions: Degenerative processes in the brain and nervous system with paralysis. Tabes. Destructive processes involving bones, periosteal pain during the night. Ulceration of skin and mucosa. Abscesses with stinking pus. Copper-coloured skin eruptions. Mental preoccupation with obsessional ideas. Fear of going mad, of incurable disease.

Mentals: Loss of memory. Lack of concentration. Not very logical thinker, bad at arithmetic. Restlessness with anxiety. Obsessive ideas with fear of infectious diseases, bacilli (compulsion to wash), paralysis, ruin, night-time (everything worse at night). Depression with suicidal tendencies.

Nervous system: Lancinating nerve pains. Headache deep down in the brain, from temple to temple; sleeplessness from midnight till 6 a.m. Ptosis of eyes. Paresis, tabes, facial paralysis. Atrophy of optic nerve.

Eyes: Pupils difffer in size. Vertical diplopia.

Ears: Caries of ossicles. Progressive deafness (otosclerosis?).

Respiratory organs: Asthma in summer, worse in warm damp weather.

CVS: Lancinating heart pain, worse at night, from base to apex. Sensation of boiling fluid in veins. Precordial pain. Vascular sclerosis. Hypertension. Angina pectoris.

Gastrointestinal: Mouth: deformed, serrated teeth. Foetor oris. Copious salivation, worse at night. Tongue: red and thick, burning, deep cracks. Ulcers in mouth, tongue, hard palate. Stomach: great desire for alcohol. Aversion to meat. Intestines: rectal strictures, ulcerations in anus, painless diarrhoea at 5 a.m., worse at seaside, anal fissures; chronic atonic constipation.

Urogenital: Induration of testes and cords. Marked fluor, thick, greenish, excoriating, worse at night. Nodular formations and ulcers in os, cervix and vulva.

Locomotor system: Pain in bones at night, particularly in long bones (tibia!). Pain at insertion of deltoid, worse at night. Back aches at night, better from movement and warmth. Juvenile kyphosis (Scheuermann's disease), bone cysts.

Skin: Copper-coloured skin eruptions. Pemphigus. Lichen planus. Foul-smelling ulceration. Abscesses with offensive smelling pus. Loss of hair in bunches or circular alopoecia.

Modalities: Worse at night; from sunset to sunrise; in summer; warmth, esp. damp warmth; thunderstorms; by the seaside. Better by day; in the mountains; walking slowly; in the cool.

Special indications: Alcoholism; addiction; moral decline; syphilis with serum reaction unchanged; children with poor capacity for logical thought, particularly if not good at arithmetic; children who do not respond to kindness nor to strictness; vicious children with outbursts of uncontrolled rage.

Summary

Thin, exhausted, restless patients who fear the nights, as all complaints get worse from sunset to sunrise. Depression with suicidal tendencies and compulsive psychotic ideas (compulsion to wash). Poor capacity for logical thought, bad at arithmetic.

Degenerative and destructive processes in nervous system and bones. Paralysis and atrophy.

Aversion to meat — a characteristic symptom in precancerous states.

TUBERCULINUM NOSODES
Nowadays we add a fourth to the three original chronic miasms: tuberculinism. The effects of this chronic infection and the profound constitutional changes it produces are very well known. Clinical experience has shown that familial disposition and constitutional factors play a role in tuberculosis. It depends on the 'soil' whether infection leads to tuberculosis or is overcome by the organism. Once again we perceive the interplay between pathogen and disposition, between heredity and environment. As Hahnemann put it, the disease is ingrained 'through infection or heredity'.

H. C. Allen referred to tuberculinism as a combination of the hereditary taints of psora and syphilis. Both components are present — the exudative, lymphatic psora element and the destructive effect of syphilis (cavities).

A number of different Tuberculinum nosodes are used, depending on the indication. The most widely used nosodes are:

1   *Tuberculinum Koch exotoxin (Tuberculinum residual)* for thin but hungry patients who are very chilly. Very prone to take cold.
2   *Tuberculinum Marmore* (French) for thin patients with poor appetite. Chilly, constipated, very nervous, dry skin.
3   *Bacillinum* if catarrhal secretions are copious, with chronic bronchitis and headache located deep down in the brain.
4   *Tuberculinum bovinum* if the symptoms are similar to those of *Tuberculinum Koch exotoxin* but milder in action.

Total picture for *Tuberculinum* nosodes:
Symptoms constantly *changing*. Changes job, address, friends, partners. Susceptible to colds, very tired, afraid of large animals (horses, cows and especially black dogs). Desire for smoked meats. Tendency to lose weight in middle life. All symptoms worse after effort, from music, change of weather, damp warm weather, draughts, in the mornings, after being asleep.

6 Use of Nosodes
With all nosodes, prescription is based on:
1   Reference to the relevant infection in the history or family history
2   Nosodes on which drug tests have been done may also be prescribed

where there is no history of the specific infection, entirely on similarity of symptoms between the presenting picture and the drug picture.

3   As intermediary drugs for patients where the best selected drug does not achieve a permanent cure and the totality of symptoms points to a specific 'miasmatic taint.'

Nosodes are therefore selected from different points of view and prescribed in different situations:

a) For the sequelae of the relevant infection if the patient has suffered from it in the past or there is a family history, e.g. positive serum reaction after treated syphilis; after inadequately treated gonorrhoea or if the mother had gonorrhoea prior to this particular pregnancy; with tuberculosis at a much earlier date in the history or frequent incidence of tuberculosis in the line of ancestors.

b) In conditions showing similarity to the drug picture of the nosode.

The conclusion to be drawn from this is that some chronic diseases show *aetiological* links to a chronic miasm (spirochaete, gonococcus, tubercle bacillus), whilst with other chronic disease processes it *seems as if* the patient had had syphilis, gonorrhoea or tuberculosis, though the history contains no evidence of such an infection. In the latter case one sees phenomenological similarity to an infection which corresponds to the drug picture of the relevant nosode. A thorough study of the drug pictures of the nosodes and their use once again illustrates Hahnemann's concept of chronic miasmatic disease as due to 'infection or heredity.' The different types of chronic disease thus serve as models for typical constitutional modes of reaction.

In a subject with latent constitutional disposition to sycotic reaction, for instance, vaccination, blood transfusions, excessive protein in the diet may *trigger* manifest sycosis with gouty or rheumatic complaints or lithiasis.

7 Diathesis

The morbid disposition arising from the constitution is referred to as 'diathesis.' The Greek verb *diatithenai* means 'to arrange.' A multiplicity of related elements is arranged in a certain order.

Having studied the drug pictures of the nosodes, a look at diathesis will provide further information to help us get a clear picture of the basic forms of chronic disease. Each of the basic chronic diseases relates to specific diatheses. Equating chronic disease and diathesis, e.g. by saying psora equals the lymphatic diathesis, would be an oversimplification. Hahnemann's chronic diseases are more comprehensive, whilst the different diatheses are more limited.

LYMPHATIC DIATHESIS

Psoric factors lead to the development of a lymphatic diathesis in childhood. This is identical with lymphatism and the exudative diathesis (Czerny). It develops the way Hahnemann has described, involving first the skin, then the mucosa and finally internal organs and systems. Milk crust, dermatitis, intertrigo, weeping eczema are often present during the first weeks of life; they are followed by coryza, bronchitis, repeated colds. Development tends to be retarded, and the child is late in learning to talk and walk. Tendency to rickets and spasmophilia. Lymphoid tissues — even normally very active in childhood — grow hypertrophic and prone to disease.

Characteristic signs of lymphatic diathesis

Skin: Exudative processes in infancy, later rough skin, poor healing tendency, with eczema, neurodermatitis, papular urticaria, urticaria, seborrhoea, intertrigo.

Lymphoid tissues: Enlarged lymph nodes in neck, axilla, inner aspect of elbow and inguinal region. Pharyngeal, palatine, submandibular tonsils, tonsillar ring.

Tongue: Papillae at tip of tongue reddened and swollen (strawberry tongue).

Nose: Blocked by lymphoid tissue and mucosal swelling. Free air passage is important for mandibular and maxillary development (dysgnathia). Mouth-breathers tend to have malpositioned teeth. Prone to develop sinusitis. 'Snotty nose'.

Eyes: Small pinhead-sized shiny nodules in mucosa of lower lid. Blepharitis.

Abdomen: Abdominal lymph nodes enlarged, sometimes palpable. Attacks of colic in infants — may lead to appendectomy when this is not indicated. Appendix is abdominal tonsil.

Bronchi: Increased mucous secretion with bronchitis, colds.

Allergic reactions: Asthma, hayfever, contact eczema, prone to infection, recurrent catarrh, pseudocroup.

Frequently indicated drugs are:
Calc.carb., Calc.phos., Calc.fluor.
Barium carb.
Silicea
Hepar sulphuris
Sulphur
Psorinum

SCROPHULOUS DIATHESIS

If there is a relatively great tuberculinic element — through infection or familial disposition — the lymphatic diathesis develops into a scrophulous diathesis. The syndrome will be unfamiliar to the younger generation of physicians, bovine tuberculosis and infection through cow's milk being very rare nowadays.

There are children who go down with recurrent and severe lymphatic reactions, usually soon after cutting their first teeth. A remarkable feature are the lips and mouth region projecting forward, like a pig's snout. Hence the name, *scropha* being the Latin for 'brood sow'. Apart from general lymphatic signs, there is often marked halitosis, increased salivation, pallid green face, high incidence of anaemia. The lymphatic drugs listed above may be indicated, and also *Merc. sol.*, *Merc. biniod*, *Tuberculinum Koch* or *Tuberculinum bovinum*.

The transition from generalized lymphatism to scrophulosis shows that the theory of miasms has its basis in reality. The tuberculin skin test is often positive in these children.

URIC ACID DIATHESIS

Within the sycotic range of constitutional disorders one often comes across the uric acid diathesis. Synonyms are lithaemic diathesis, rheumatic-gouty diathesis, hydrogenoid diathesis (v. Grauvogl).

Characteristic features are:
— Rheumatic conditions affecting joints, muscles, tendons, nerves (neuritis)
— Gouty deposits in joints, tendons and especially the basal joints of the great toe and thumb, Achilles tendon, outer ear (tophi)
— Concretions in the urogenital system (urates), inflammatory conditions in the urogenital region
— Liver and gallbladder disease, concretions in bile ducts
— Metabolic disorders with hyperuricaemia, hypercholesterolaemia, hyperlipaemia, diabetes and consequently increased risk of arteriosclerosis and cardiovascular disease
— Benign tumours ranging from warts to fibroids, adenomas (prostate) and uterine myomas.
    Symptoms are usually worse in cold damp weather; humid climates, particularly by inland waters (but not at the seaside!); in narrow river valleys; from cold water applications; cold baths; sequelae of vaccinations.

Frequently indicated drugs:
        Thuja   Sarsaparilla

Natrum sulphuricum	Lithium carbonicum
Acidum nitricum	*Rhus toxicodendron*
Lycopodium	*Colchicum*
Berberis	*Dulcamara*
Acidum benzoicum	*Urtica urens*
Acidum formicum	*Adlumina fung.*
Antimonium crudum	*Medorrhinum*

DYSCRATIC DIATHESIS

The dyscratic diathesis belongs to the syphilinic range of constitutional disorders. In humoral pathology, the term dyscrasia was used to define a depraved state of the humours, a state of imbalance.

This diathesis is less clearly defined than the others as it relates to the end states of processes arising through psoric, sycotic and above all also tuberculinic taints.

The diathesis often provides the background for the development of carcinomas and other malignant tumours and malignant blood disease (leukaemia a.o.).

Degenerative diseases of the nervous system such as tabes and paralysis may also be considered to come under this heading.

Frequently indicated drugs:

Acidum nitricum	Heavy metals:	*Aurum*
Arsenicum album		*Plumbum*
Carbo animalis		*Thallium*
Hydrastis		*Mercurius*
Iodum		
Kalium bichromicum	Nosode:	*Syphilinum*
Kalium iodatum		
Kreosotum		
Silicea		

8 Review of the Basic Types of Chronic Disease

A study of the drug pictures of the nosodes, comparing them with the relevant diatheses and chronic infections, provides us with an overview of the directions in which congenital or acquired constitutional taints may evolve to give rise to chronic disease.

Table 12 gives the characteristic signs and symptoms of psora, sycosis, syphilis and tuberculinism.[18]

Tabular presentation makes it possible to consider each form on its own, moving down the relevant column, or to compare all four side by side. Comparison is important, for it shows that these are not pathological units but constitutional differences in reaction. Such dispositions based on constitution are rarely seen in their pure form; mixed forms with one element predominating are much more common. Life is always in a state of flux and the borders between the different types are therefore fluid.

Psoric conditions are most common in young people, the middle years are often marked by sycotic processes, and in old age these change to syphilinic degeneration. Synoptic comparison will help to overcome a static view of rigidly defined disease states and encourage us to think in terms of dynamic disease processes.

CHARACTERISTIC REACTIONS

Hahnemann's chronic diseases define basic types of physical and emotional imbalance. Health may be defined as a balanced 'steady state' of all vital processes (von Berthalanffy), the individual being in harmony with himself, his environment and creation.

This defines disease as a deviation from being in harmony and adapted to internal, external and cosmic conditions.

Hahnemann's theory of chronic disease indicated three directions in which functional and structural deviation may go. The three directions are discernible among the multiplicity of disorders shown in the synopsis if major trends are looked for and determined. These may be summarized as follows:

Physical Reactions
Psora represents functional weakness
Hypotrophy, hypotension
Basic principle: Deficiency
The deficiency state is due to inadequate utilization in the mineral metabolism. The parents, grandparents etc. of these patients often show the same drug constitution, as Mezger was able to demonstrate in the case of *Magnesium* (see p. 186). The family history also shows a relatively high incidence of allergic disease and lymphatic diatheses. Suppression should be looked for in the patient's history. Suppression of skin eruptions (*Sulphur!*) and physiological eliminations (sweat, menses, diarrhoea) activates the particular disposition to react which is inherent in the constitution. Skin eruptions then shift to respiratory disorders or gastrointestinal disease.

Sycosis — Humoral imbalance leads to deposits and proliferations
Hypertrophy, hypertension

Basic principle: Excess
Here parents, grandparents etc. frequently suffered from metabolic disorders (gout, rheumatism, renal and biliary concretions, raised cholesterol levels, arteriosclerosis). The sycotic mode of reaction is provoked by gonorrhoea, chronic pelvic inflammations, cumulative sequelae of vaccination, injections of foreign protein, excessive food intake, especially protein and carbohydrates, blood transfusions. Suppression of pathological eliminations (e.g. fluor, nasal secretions) and proliferations (warts, cysts, fibroids) frequently leads to the manifestation of sycosis.

Syphilis — Organic lesions with ulceration and tissue destruction Dystrophy, dystonia
Basic principle: Destruction
Family history of malignant tumours, blood disease, degenerative nervous disease, pyschosis, alcoholism, high incidence of suicide. Congenital and acquired syphilis will trigger this mode of reaction, and so will neurotropic virus diseases (herpes viruses, slow virus

Table 11: Synopsis of Mental and Emotional Reactions

	Psora	Sycosis	Syphilis
Principal characteristic	unassuming	exaggerated	aggressive
Extremes of range from-to	active, enthusiastic — inhibited, fearful	powerful, over-weening — chaotic, confused	dictatorial — silly
	communicative — reserved	euphoric — distrustful	apathetic — violent
Character	weakly, sparse, inadequate	boasting, intrusive	nervous, spiteful
	anxious, shy, pusillanimous	overrating him- or herself, demanding	destructive, aimless
	mean, pedantic	unsettled, busy	suicide
Tendency	yearning	adaptation	revolution
Colour preference	blue	yellow	red
Clothes	neutral, tidy	garish, exaggerated	untidy, disreputable
	out of fashion	latest fashion	slovenly
Pathological range	inferiority complexes	fixed ideas, scruples	guilt complexes, compulsive actions
	anxiety syndromes	neurosis	psychosis

Sources: Allen HC, Dorcsi M, Mueller HV, Speight Ph.

infections). Suppression of pathological eliminations, of ulcers and tumours may enhance the syphilinic reaction.

Mental and Emotional Reactions
Soma and psyche are different facets of the ensouled body. The mental and emotional state of a person corresponds to somatic deviations. In this sphere, too, three degrees of miasmatic taint are discernible. This takes us to a deeper level of Hahnemann's concept of disordered vital energies, the latter being a non-physical entity. Here we are given an indication, for ourselves and for our patients, each for himself and his own way of life, of a proper mode of life. *Disorder in the non-physical vital energies first comes to expression in wrong thinking, progressing through wrong intentions to wrong actions.*

Homoeopathic history-taking (*Organon* §§ 83-104) penetrates to this, the deepest level of human ill-health. Through the medical biography it traces the first beginnings of wrong thinking and wrong intentions.

Whichever level we start at, the aim is always to find the appropriate drug. This is the essential difference from psychoanalytical therapy. The homoeopathic drug relates to features discernible in psyche and soma. In establishing the mental and emotional reactions relating to the three basic types of chronic disease, it is important to perceive also the corresponding somatic features, including them for the purposes of drug diagnosis.

9 Treatment Scheme for Chronic Diseases

OBSTACLES

1   *Removal of foci.* It is important not to become obsessed with foci. The similar drug will often give a cure in spite of foci being present. Foci will often react to drug therapy and make themselves felt. Obvious dental foci should be dealth with. Preliminary treatment with *Arnica* 6c (12x), 8 drops daily for 3-5 days.

Surgical scars may be treated by injecting 0.5% xylocaine beneath; tonsillectomy scars. Chronically infected tonsils — vacuum removal of pus may be indicated (Roeder method). In case of doubt consult colleagues with specialist experience in detection of foci and neural therapy.

2   *Actions and sequelae of allopathic drugs.* If absolutely necessary, allow present treatment to continue. If medically justifiable reduce dosage gradually until able to discontinue. Medication should not be stopped abruptly. In making the homoeopathic drug diagnosis it

Table 12: Synopsis of Symptoms and Signs

Psora	Sycosis	Syphilis	Tuberculinism (psora + syphilis)
	Principal action		
Functional disorders Neurovegetative imbalances Endocrine disorders Skin, mucosa, lymphoid tissue react strongly	*Excessive tissue reaction* in connective tissue, muscles, tendons: rheumatic complaints; benign growths, cysts, warts in skin and mucosa Concretions in kidneys and gall-bladder	*Tissue destruction* nerve tissue: paralysis; skin: deep ulceration, fissures, destructive suppuration; all organs: destruction Affecting mainly nervous system, bones, glands	*Marked lymphatic reaction and destruction* primary tubercular affect becomes destructive cheesy suppuration, cavitation Affecting mainly lymph glands, lungs, bones, liver adrenals
		Physiognomy	
Facies Pale, earth-coloured, as if unwashed Skin dry, rough, pimply, often yellow Very pale during first sleep Red and transparent if febrile	Pale, pallid, thickened skin, large pores, orange-peel skin, greasy, shiny Face sweating Red nose, with enlarged capillaries	Greasy, smeary, grey, as if emaciated Midface regressing High cheekbones	Thin skin, veins visible on pink or bluish background, waxy Red patches if febrile
	Warts, fibromas, papillomas	Copper-coloured patches Papillomas	
	Red patches, esp. cheekbones and below eyes		
Lips red	Thickened lips	Thickened lips	Thickened lips — extremely red, as if blood would spurt from them Bulging upper lip: scrophula Fissures

	Psora	Sycosis	Syphilis	Tuberculinism (psora + syphilis)
Eyes	Inflamed lids	Sparse lashes	Eyebrows and lashes irregular	Wide pupils Lid margins red Granulomatous inflammation of lid margins Long lashes
Hair	Dry, lustreless, dull, early greyness, rough		Dry as hemp or oily, greasy	Dry like tow, or damp, matted

Suppressions encourage development of the latent morbidity and shift the balance from harmless local maladies to serious organic disease. Every diathesis has a point where it is particularly open to attack and reacts to suppression in a characteristic way.

	Psora	Sycosis	Syphilis	Tuberculinism (psora + syphilis)
Nature and location of suppressed element	Skin eruptions Physiological eliminations: sweat, stools, urine, menses	Pathological eliminations: fluor, nasal and aural secretions Surgical removal of warts, fistulas, fibromas, myomas	Pathological eliminations: fistulas, ulceration, suppuration	Skin eruptions Normal and pathological eliminations (see under psora and syphilis) Particularly suppression of sweating of feet
Consequences of suppression	Nervous and mental symptoms	Diseases of pelvic and sexual organs: inflammation, hypertrophy, abscesses, cysts Headaches, psychotic states	Diseases affecting meninges, paralysis Larynx, eyes, bones	Headaches States of excitement Suppuration Cavitation

Modalities

Triggered or aggravated by suppression of normal and pathological eliminations

Psora	Sycosis	Syphilis	Tuberculinism (psora + syphilis)
Worse from			
Standing, movement	Rest		Forceful movement
Mental excitement: worry, grief, fear, anxiety	Mental excitement		Excitement (as for psora)
Anger causes sadness	Anger causes violent reaction	Anger causes violent reaction	Physical and mental effort, mountain climbing
Time:	Time:		
mornings	after midnight, esp. early hours (except for *Med*)	sunset to sunrise	at night
Pain comes and goes with the sun			
Sunlight (eyes)	Artificial light		Artificial light
Before menses	Any change in weather	Gales	
Strong smells	Weather damp, steamy, and damp and cold	Great cold and heat (generally)	
Noise	After sweats, stools	By the seaside	
		In winter	
		Sweating a great deal	
Better from			
Lying down	Prone position	Movement	Distraction, travel (esp. mental symptoms)
Rest	Slow movement	In the mountains	Local heat ameliorates pain
Quiet	Dry weather	Cold applications (if in pain)	
Warmth (if in pain)			Temporary relief from outbreak of sweat, esp. on feet
Physiological eliminations: sweat, stools, urine	Reappearance of menses or suppressed physiological eliminations	Old ulceration recurring, ulcer becoming open, old inflammation	

Psora	Sycosis	Syphilis	Tuberculinism (psora + syphilis)
Mental conditions improved if physical illness develops	Pathological eliminations bring rapid improvement: fluor, catarrh, outbreak of warts, development of fibromas		Mental symptoms better once old ulcer breaks out again
		General symptoms	
Rapid alternation of all symptoms	Very slow convalescence	Delayed healing tendency	Rapid alternation of mental and physical symptoms
	Repeated relapses	Often only minimal prodomal signs before organic changes manifest	Nocturnal sweats give temporary relief
Dryness	Very gradual progression	Heavy sweats exhaust, with no relief	
Hot flushes	Febrile reaction rare	Rapid weight loss, looks emaciated	
Conscious of pulsations		Boring bone pain worse at night	
Burning hands and feet			
Eliminations thin, watery, acrid	Eliminations jelly-like	Eliminations acrid and foul-smelling	
	Stiff and lame	Restless if in pain, has to keep moving	

Psora	Sycosis	Syphilis	Tuberculinism (psora + syphilis)
Symptoms are intensely experienced and frequently described in 'as if' terms Many concomitant symptoms Strange foods desired Capricious in desires and aversions Hunger with debility or aversion to food, to milk		Aversion to meat	Desire for cold milk and alcohol Great hunger
		Local symptoms	
Head Headache: mostly frontal, temporal, lateral	vertex	base of skull or hemicrania	often on rest days
Worse in morning, or increasing and decreasing as sun rises and goes down, from sun's rays, cold	Worse at night, at or after midnight Early hours of morning Lying down Physical or mental effort	Worse at night, resting, lying down, from warmth	Worse from nervous excitement, preparing for examinations
Better from warmth, rest or sleep, quiet	Better from movement	Better towards morning, from cold, movement, epistaxis Sensation of band	Better from eating, epistaxis Sensation of band

Psora	Sycosis	Syphilis	Tuberculinism (psora + syphilis)
	Often accompanied with restlessness, febrile sensation, coldness of body, exhaustion	Often accompanied with vertigo, pushes head into pillow or rolls head to and fro	Accompanied with rush of blood to head and chest, hot or cold hands and feet, great exhaustion and despondency
			Often prodomal hunger
		Tends to persist for days	Tends to persist for days
			Very severe headache
Scalp and hair			
Dry eruptions with marked irritation, worse in open air			Moist eruptions with marked irritation
Scratching causes burning pain			Thick crusts of dried pus
White dandruff			
Head sweats easily			
Alopoecia, esp. following acute illness	Alopoecia areata (circular)	Alopoecia in bunches or patches (circular)	Alopoecia following headache or febrile illness
Premature greying or greying in patches			Hair smells like stale hay
Hair breaking or splitting	Hair smelling sour or fishy	Hair smelling sour or putrid	Damp, matted, oily and greasy, or dry like tow or hemp
Likes head covered			Likes head covered

Psora	Sycosis	Syphilis	Tuberculinism (psora + syphilis)
Eyes			
Affected parts: conjunctiva, lid margins. With sensation of burning and dryness	Marked blepharitis with thick, yellowy-green secretions	Major refractory anomalies	Refractory anomalies
	Corneal inflammation — superficial ulcers	Deep ulceration and specific inflammation	Ulceration and specific inflammation of sclera, iris, cornea and tear ducts
		Degenerative processes and inflammation of sclera, iris	
		Optic nerve atrophy	
Sensitive to daylight, less so to artificial light	Sensitive to artificial light	Sensitive to artificial light	
Inflammation usually better from warmth			Exanthematous childhood diseases cause serious eye inflammations
Ears			
Hypersensitive to noise		Many organic diseases of the ear.	Many organic diseases of the ear, esp. following febrile illnesses or exanthematous childhood diseases (esp. measles and scarlet fever)
Meatus dry and itching			Severe otitis media, with destruction of bone tissue
			Pus smelling of old cheese, often crumbly texture

Psora	Sycosis	Syphilis	Tuberculinism (psora + syphilis)
Nose			Least chill causes nocturnal otalgia
Hypersensitive to all smells	Loss of sense of smell	Loss of sense of smell	Weeping eczema, fissures, crusts around and esp. behind ear
Smells cause headache, nausea and vertigo	Coryza thin, watery, acrid		Excessive epistaxis following heat or effort, at the least occasion
Epistaxis	Sensation: hot, burning	Hayfever of extreme severity	Blood in catarrhal and hayfever secretions
Sensation of dryness in nose	Hayfever with rapid alternation between being blocked and unblocked	Ulceration	Yellowy coryza smelling of old cheese or sulphuretted hydrogen
	Greeny yellow pus smelling of fish	Thick crusts, dark or greenish secretions	Retrograde secretion
	Copious thin mucus in cold winds	Snuffling a great deal	
		Destruction of nasal bone tissue	
Mouth			Lips extremely red, fissures
Lips red, swollen, burning, dry		Tonsils enlarged	Tonsils enlarged
Bitter, sweetish, sour taste in mouth		Position of teeth irregular	Position of teeth irregular
Protracted after-taste of food		Teeth deformed, serrated	Mouth ulcers
			Deep ulcers

Psora	Sycosis	Syphilis	Tuberculinism (psora + syphilis)
Sense of taste distorted: bread tastes bitter, water putrid		Teeth converge towards tip Caries at gingival margins, teeth break off before fully developed Deep gingival ulcers Metallic taste in mouth Marked salivation, viscous, tastes of metal or copper	Gums bleed a great deal Caries before teeth have developed Eruption of teeth very painful, with diarrhoea and fever Metallic taste in mouth, or of pus or blood, or putrid
Stomach Foods desired: sweet, sugar, hot, sour, tasty, tea, coffee, tobacco, hot dishes; pregnant women and children: indigestible items	beer, roast meats, rich foods, well seasoned; hot or cold dishes Food combustion inadequate, resulting in tissue deposits and concretions Rich foods and meats enhance sycotic phenomena Aversion to onions Gastric pain, better lying prone or from pressure, from movement Cramp-like, colicky pain	cold dishes	children: indigestible foods; salt; cold foods and drinks; stimulants: beer, wine, meat, potatoes, tea, coffee, tobacco
Aversion to cooked foods		Aversion to meat	Aversion to fats common

Psora	Sycosis	Syphilis	Tuberculinism (psora + syphilis)
Appetite			Exhausted unless hunger is satisfied
Unnatural hunger at unusual times, incl. at night			Eat more than able to cope with
Hunger, feels very debilitated			No appetite in the mornings, but hunger at other times
Hunger, feels full after a few mouthfuls			
or: ravenous hunger must eat immediately or feels faint			
sweats when eating			
Hunger at 11 a.m.			
Fullness and gases forming after eating			
Sour or bitter eructations			
Desire to sleep after meals			
Abdomen			
Feels full after meals	Frequent colics		Frequent chronic constipation
Pressure in liver region	Better on movement, firm pressure, lying prone		Diarrhoea with cold sweats
Sensation as if intestines hanging down	Colicky diarrhoea with mucus and great irritability	Nocturnal diarrhoea with hot or cold sweat and marked exhaustion	Diarrhoea after milk, from cold, when teething
Rumbling and gurgling in gut, worse after milk, from cold water, potatoes, beans			Diarrhoea with mucus or blood
			Great exhaustion after diarrhoea
			Stools grey, lacking in bile

Psora	Sycosis	Syphilis	Tuberculinism (psora + syphilis)
Colis or diarrhoea from getting chilled Pain better from warmth or very gentle pressure Frequent chronic constipation Diarrhoea from overeating, from cold, often worse in the mornings (Podophyllum, Aloe, Sulphur) Diarrhoea due to mental or emotional factors Alternating constipation and diarrhoea Diarrhoea exhausts	Rectum: fissures, strictures, bleeding haemorrhoids with thin secretions smelling of fish		Rectum: fistulas, strictures, fissures Rectal disease alternating with cardiac or pulmonary disease Surgical treatment for haemorrhoids may trigger asthma or cardiac disease
Respiratory organs No organic changes Dry spasmodic cough	Cough producing only small amount of clear mucus Cough in autumn and winter, better in summer		Deep cough with purulent or mucopurulent expectoration, tasting sweetish or salty

Psora	Sycosis	Syphilis	Tuberculinism (psora + syphilis)
	Cough following slightest chill Nasal breathing poor Bronchitis starts with cough which goes down to chest		Expectoration may be bloody Cough exhausts Worse at night Respiration impeded, superficial breathing Abdominal breathing poor
Heart Functional heart disease with anxiety, sharp, cutting pain Heart symptoms after fear, loss, excessive joy, after meals, often worse Nocturnal palpitations when lying supine	Valve defects, myocardial lesions Relatively little anxiety or pain with heart conditions Soft, slow pulse	patients die suddenly, with no prior warning Sycotic and syphilitic organic heart disease tends to be serious, but is not experienced as such	Heart symptoms usually have hypotensive character, with states of collapse Worse from effort Better lying down Cannot climb mountains Blood drained from head at high altitudes
Urinary system Ischuria after chill or in consequence of reflectory disorders due to other diseases, esp. in abdomen and female genitalia Involuntary miction after sneezing, coughing, laughing	Cramp-like pain in urethra and bladder Children cry when voiding Concretions in kidney and bladder Gouty kidney Nephritis	Febrilenephritis	Urine smells of stale hay or like rotten meat Enuresis during first sleep

Psora	Sycosis	Syphilis	Tuberculinism (psora + syphilis)
White, yellow or rust-coloured sediment if febrile, phosphaturia			
Genital organs			
Functional disease	Colicky pain with menses, in bouts		Menses exhausting, prolonged and heavy, bright red, too early, often with vertigo, debility, headache, diarrhoea, epistasis
Periods too short or interrupted, or too heavy or too light, rarely normal	Fluor heavy, acrid, excoriating, with fishy smell		Anxious mentality, irritable, at the same time weepy
Dysmenorrhoea common in puberty	Menses often burning, excoriating		Fluor purulent or thin and viscous or thick and yellow, yellow green
Sharp pain	Pelvic inflammation, esp. female genitalia		Uterus often retroflexed
	Cysts in ovaries, tubes, uterus		Parturition tends to be difficult
	Appendicitis		Breast-feeding usually not possible
			Hydrocoele
			Prostatitis with exhausting involuntary discharge of secretions or seminal fluid
Extremities			
Neuralgic pain, better if resting, lying down, from warmth	Stiff and lame	Diseases of bone and periosteum, lymph glands	Diseases of bone
Leg cramps	Worse in initial stages of movement, bending down		Rickets
Hands and feet dry and hot	Shooting, tearing pain	Stabbing, shooting, boring pain	Bones soft and bent
			Pain as with syphilis

Psora	Sycosis	Syphilis	Tuberculinism (psora + syphilis)
Burning sensation in palms and soles	Worse resting, when barometer is falling, in warm and in cold, damp weather, storms	Worse at night or in early part of night, in cold and damp weather	Paronychia in pale, anaemic subjects
Numbness, pins and needles in hands at least pressure	Better from rubbing and stretching, dry weather		Nails break or split easily
Sensation of coldness in individual parts: knee, hand, also nose and ear	Gouty deposits		Fingers very long
	Calcareous deposits around joints		Longitudinal proportions of fingers irregular
	Rheumatic deformation		Narrow hands, soft
	Nails often furrowed or ridged		Hands or feet damp, sweating easily or cold
Able to walk well, but not to stand	Paralysis — oedema — swelling	Paralysis — odema — swelling	Generalized muscular weakness
	Striae on thigh		Lack of co-ordination when moving, falls easily or lets things drop
	Cellulitis		Joints turn over easily, sprains
			Connective tissue weakness
			Pain and swelling after playing piano, typing
Skin			
Dry, rough, as if unwashed	Greasy, smeary, oily, blotched		Delicate, transparent skin
	Warts, fibromas, red naevi		Damp, increased perspiration, rarely reduced perspiration
	Tendency for striae, cellulitis		Tendency for freckles

Psora	Sycosis	Syphilis	*Tuberculinism* (psora + syphilis)
Skin eruptions very irritating, burning if scratched, worse late evening till midnight	Skin eruptions: irregular scales in circumscribed patches	Skin eruptions around joints, in flexures, ring-shaped, copper-coloured or like raw ham or brownish, may be very red at base, no irritation	Pustular eczema
Skin eruptions with small vesicles, like scabies	Eczemas with loss of epidermal tissue (exfoliative eczema)	Thick scales and crusts, circular	Herpes, urticaria, abscesses
Minimal pus formation, usually only seropurulent or blood-stained secretions	Tinea barbae, herpes zoster	Proliferations, crested growths (cockscomb)	Ulcerations, impetigo
Micropapular eczema	Pedunculated warts, smooth warts, condylomas, acuminate warts	Pemphigoid skin eruptions	Insect bites provoke powerful reactions
Thin scales and crusts	Acne, very sensitive to touch	Copper-coloured patches turning blue in the cold	Varicosities and varicose ulcers
	Worse around time of menses		Purpura, ecchymoses
	Varicella		Lupus (usually in conjunction with sycosis and psora)
	Smallpox vaccination enhances sycotic symptoms (sometimes also syphilitic symptoms)		
	Erysipelas		
	Impetigo		
	Spider naevi in face, esp. below eyes or on cheek bones		
	Poor postoperative wound healing		

Psora	Sycosis	Syphilis	Tuberculinism (psora + syphilis)
	Symptoms relating to mind and intellect		
Quick-minded, mentally active, lively	Irritable, cross, morose	Heavy, slow	Initially hyperactive, quickly exhausts himself, no staying power
Impressible, exhausted following emotional strain	Distrusts others and even self	Indolent	Erratic, loses thread, does not take things in
Exalted	Jealous	Dull	Unsociable, shut themselves off and grow morose
Likes to express feelings, communicative	Keeps things to himself	Simple, dull-witted	Real problem children
	Makes a mystery of quite unimportant things	Apathetic, indifferent	
		Stiff-necked, self-willed, obstinate	Failure at school
		Withdrawn, tight-lipped, do not communicate	Like change of location, job, partner
Vexation causes sadness	Vexation provokes violent reactions	Slow on the uptake, thoughts vanish, cannot get them together	
Nervous, fearful, restless	Likes to repeat himself when writing or speaking	Vexation provokes violent reactions	
Poor concentration	Tends to brood		
Absent, forgetful, jumps from point to point when talking	Forgets words, cannot find the right words	Logical thinking poor	
	Poor orthography	Bad at arithmetic	
	Forgets, things of immediate concern, remembers past things well		

Psora	Sycosis	Syphilis	Tuberculinism (psora + syphilis)
Mentals	Self-condemnation Fixed ideas: body fragile	Definite guilt complexes Fixed ideas: fear of infectious diseases, of germs (compulsion to wash) Depressed, melancholic: but will not talk about it	
Suicide uncommon	High incidence of suicide	Suicide committed unexpectedly	
Better with all physiological eliminations: sweat, diarrhoea, powerful diuresis and reappearance of old, suppressed skin eruptions	Better with increased pathological eliminations: fluor, catarrhal secretions, esp. if previously suppressed Better if warts form	Better with increased pathological eliminations, fluor, catarrhal secretions, esp. if previously suppressed	Temporarily better following increased body, axillary or foot sweat, boil opening up Worse if foot sweats suppressed Suppressed foot sweats induce mental symptoms and also organic lesions

is often difficult to say which symptoms are side effects of allopathic drugs and which form part of the individual disease picture. *Nux vomica* 4x or *Sulphur* 6c (12x) may help to clarify the situation.

3   *Look for consequences of suppression.* A major fact which has emerged from Hahnemann's researches is that the suppression of skin eruptions and physiological eliminations (sweat, secretions, menses) or pathological secretions (from nose, throat, vagina, urethra, anus) runs counter to nature's healing efforts.

   Sulphur is a major drug for treating the sequelae of suppression, but not the only one.

(Consult the relevant rubrics in Kent:
E.g. Head, Pain, following suppression
suppressed eruptions — p. 149
coryza, suppressed, from having a — p. 138
menses, during, suppressed — p. 142
perspiration, suppressed, from — p. 145
general consequences of suppressed fever (= quinine, abuse of) — p. 1397)

SUPPORTIVE MEASURES

It is obviously important to advise a balanced diet and life style, again on an individual basis, depending on the modalities in each case. Coffee, tea, alcohol and tobacco may possibly be permitted in moderate amounts. Herbal teas made with medicinal herbs, especially chamomile, should not be permitted. The diet should be low in acids, except for foods containing lactic acid; citrus fruits need to be limited. Meat from fattened animals and pork to be avoided.

Hahnemann's rules relating to diet and life style were stringent (*Chronic Diseases* vol. 1, pp. 134-144 in the German original, and §§ 259 and 260 in the *Organon*). He no doubt had good reasons for this, but it has to be admitted that in the present age they are not adhered to in absolutely every point. We have to use a certain restraint in imposing restrictions. The concurrent use of 'household remedies' is fairly easily stopped by referring to their cost. People will respond to financial arguments where they do not listen to reason. Toothpaste should not be used before and after taking a homoeopathic drug; instead, the teeth should be cleaned by brushing with water only.

Holiday plans and visits to health resorts should fit into the context. The seaside is not the best place for everyone, nor does everyone find the mountains the best place for a holiday. (See e.g. Kent's *Repertory*: Mind, high places agg. — p. 51; bathing, sea, agg. — p. 1346; bathing, agg. 1345; air, seashore, agg. p. 1344. Generally better in the mountains: *Syphilinum*.)

A warm-hearted and optimistic approach on the practitioner's part will help the patient to a more positive attitude; guidance is a skill which can be acquired. Chronic patients have usually had so many negative experiences that the contribution made by the physician's personality to the healing process is negligible. It is better to put our trust in the similar drug rather than charisma.

DRUG DIAGNOSIS
Full case-taking is a precondition, and a careful clinical diagnosis should be a matter of course.

Table 13 summarizes the chapter on case-taking and the preceding sections. The similar drug chosen in a case of chronic illness must correspond to the totality of presenting and biographical symptoms and signs.

The *peculiar* (§ 153) shows itself in the symptoms of the *present* stage of the disease; what is *characteristic* is the sequence of recurring disorders the particular nature of which may be discerned from the past history. The basic disorder (psora, sycosis, syphilis, tuberculinism) may be discernible as a uniform constitutional background to the multiplicity of symptoms found in the past history.

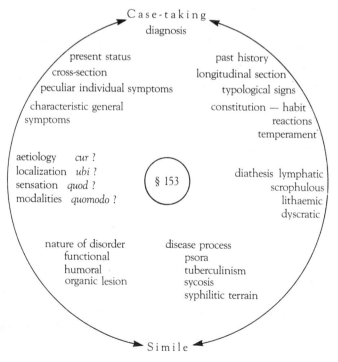

Case-taking
diagnosis

present status   past history
cross-section   longitudinal section
peculiar individual symptoms   typological signs
characteristic general   constitution — habit
symptoms   reactions
                                                    temperament

aetiology   *cur ?*   diathesis lymphatic
localization *ubi ?*   § 153   scrophulous
sensation   *quod ?*   lithaemic
modalities   *quomodo ?*   dyscratic

nature of disorder   disease process
functional   psora
humoral   tuberculinism
organic lesion   sycosis
                                syphilitic terrain

S i m i l e

'The presenting disease needs to be seen as part of the total biographical existence of the patient, and we must be clearly aware that the presenting pathological phenomena arise out of a whole and converge in a whole.'[19]

SEQUENCE OF DRUGS

Psora, sycosis or syphilis rarely occur in their pure forms. Because of this, it is often necessary to consider a number of drugs in making the final choice. If the drug diagnosis is uncertain at first and the choice an open one, the decision is based on the following sequence:

— plants
— nosodes
— mineral salts
— metals

If the drugs in question relate to a number of different constitutional defects or if the basic disorder cannot be clearly discerned, the sequence is:

— psora
— tuberculinism
— sycosis
— syphilis

EUGENIC THERAPY

Eugenic therapy, a prophylactic measure for the benefit of the child developing in utero, uses the same sequence, all other constitutional defects having developed on the basis of psora.

Method: a single dose of the drug is given, always at intervals of one week; the 30c potency is used as it corresponds most closely to the maternal constitution.

1st week: a psoric drug
           (*Sulphur, Calcarea, Magnesium* a.o.)
2nd week: a tuberculinic nosode
           (*Tuberculinum Koch* or *bovinum* a.o.)
3rd week: a sycotic drug
           (*Thuja* or *Natrum sulph., Medorrhinum* a.o.)
4th week: *Syphilinum*

The course of treatment should be given as early as possible, ideally during the first 3 months of pregnancy.

AVOIDABLE ERRORS

1   Lack of patience is a cardinal error, and 'in the treatment of chronic diseases homoeopathic physicians need to take extreme care and be most persevering in avoiding it'. 'If we reflect on the great

changes which the drug must effect in many, incredibly subtle parts of the living organism in order to eradicate this kind of deep-rooted chronic miasm and restore a state of health . . . '

The action of a drug given in high potency persists for a very long time 'and must not . . . be disrupted or cancelled by a new drug'.[20]

It is therefore important to give the drug time to take full effect. The same drug should be given at long intervals in *different* potencies for a period of many months. Do not change the drug unless absolutely convinced that the disease picture has changed.

2   Lack of conviction.

If we prescribe one thing today and another tomorrow, using a new drug to deal with every minor problem the patient presents, we shall never reach our goal.

A stomach upset will respond well to a day's fasting, a chill to rising footbaths (caution with varicose veins!), and a chest pack will often cure a developing cough. When a patient complains of new symptoms we should first of all consider if this is not a necessary crisis of elimination (skin, gut, kidneys). Psoric disorders are better from increased physiological elimination (sweat, urine, stools, menses), particularly if these have previously been suppressed. Sycotic and syphilinic conditions improve with increased pathological eliminations.

Degenerative conditions cannot be cured unless inflammation develops.

If it proves impossible to manage an intercurrent acute condition without drug therapy, plant-based drugs should be given preference, e.g. sudden fright — *Opium*; anger, with serious upset — *Chamomilla*; distress — *Ignatia*; jealousy — *Hyoscyamus*; diarrhoea due to chill — *Dulcamara*, etc.

10 Summary

Hahnemann's *Chronic Diseases* provides a magnificent basic theory which is critically assessed, deepened and developed further in the light of present-day knowledge.

Some of his theoretical expositions are time-bound and therefore limited. This does not, however, reflect on the genuine merit of his work which is as important today as it was in his time: to find and test the drugs which prove effective and define their range of action.

The essentials may be summarized as follows:

1   Prescriptions should not be based on the presenting picture only; the totality of symptoms includes the history and family history.

We must treat the patient, not the disease.

2   Chronic diseases have a character of their own. Their symptoms increase in number in the course of life. Vital energies are unable to overcome them on their own. Even a perfectly balanced diet and life style make no essential difference. A cure is possible only through the homoeopathic drug which matches the whole of the underlying disorder.

3   This basic underlying disorder has arisen 'through heredity or infection'; Hahnemann refers to it by the term 'miasm' which was common medical usage from the time of Hippocrates to his own.

   Constitutional genetic defects and acquired infection change the reactivity of the vital force which is responsible for central regulation. Hahnemann was the first to speak of the way chronic infection had a negative effect on constitution, long before bacteriology (Koch) appeared on the scene.

4   Hahnemann classified chronic diseases in three groups which he named after the characteristic skin changes occurring in the initial stage:

   — Scabies (the itch) = psora; skin eruptions causing the patient to scratch
   — Condylomas = sycosis; proliferative skin and mucosal changes
   — Chancres = syphilis (nowadays 'syphilinic conditions'); ulceration and tissue breakdown, ulcers in skin and mucosa

   These skin and mucosal changes serve to relieve the system. Suppression causes the rapid spread of the underlying internal disorder.

   It is therefore important to avoid all forms of external suppression.

   The internal disease needs to be treated with the appropriate durg.

5   Today we no longer subscribe to Hahnemann's unicausal theory and instead classify chronic diseases according to the total symptomatology of corresponding disease models: disorders of mineral metabolism, gonorrhoea, syphilis.

   Drug pictures of the nosodes *Psorinum*, *Medorrhinum* and *Syphilinum*

   Drug pictures of the principal drugs *Sulphur*, *Thuja* and *Mercury*

   Diathesis — lymphatic, gouty/rheumatic/lithaemic, dyscratic

   The three basic forms of chronic disease are therefore seen as models for particular modes of pathological reaction and constitutional defects in patients with chronic disease.

6   Drug diagnosis takes its orientation from characteristic general symptoms and peculiar individual symptoms in the presenting condition and also from the typological signs of the chronic disorder evident from the history.

7   If treatment proves unsuccessful, potential obstacles must be looked for — foci of infection, sequelae of allopathic treatment or suppression, faulty life style.

8   Patience and confidence in one's approach to treatment are essential preconditions if success is to be achieved.

[1]   *Chronic Diseases*, p. 4 of German original.

[2]   ibid., p. 6 of German original.

[3]   ibid., pp. 6-7 of German original.

[4]   Imhaeuser [1970] p. 144. I have seen very good results with hayfever.

[5]   *Chronic Diseases*, p. 11 of German original.

[6]   ibid., p. 6 of German original.

[7]   ibid., p. 51 of German original.

[8]   ibid., p. 105 of German original.

[9]   ibid., p. 8 of German original.

[10]   ibid., pp. 11-12 of German original.

[11]   See Gebser, *Ursprung und Gegenwart*, quoting Pascal: 'You would not have been looking for me unless you had already found me.'

[12]   Quoted from Bier, *Homoeopathie und harmonische Ordnung der Heilkunde* [1949], p. 221.

[13]   ibid., p. 222.

[14]   Mezger [1951], p. 509.

[15]   Quoted from Voegeli [1961], p. 74.

[16]   Quoted from Mezger [1951], p. 400.

[17]   For detailed drug pictures of the nosodes, see Julian AO, *Materia medica der Nosoden* (Engl. also *Practical materia medica of biotherapies and nosodes*, trs. R. Mulserji. New Delhi: B. Jain 1980).

[18]   It was the work of Ph. Speight which encouraged me to compile a synopsis. The whole is based on the following sources: Hahnemann's *Chronic Diseases*; Allen TF, *The Chronic Miasms*; Dorcsi, *Stufenplan und Ausbildungsprogramm*; Hind, Jai (ed.), *Chronic Diseases and Theory of Miasms*; Fortier-Bernoville, *Syphilis and Sycosis*; Voegeli A, *Die rheumatischen Erkrankungen*. Ortega's forthcoming publication *Bemerkungen zu Hahnemanns Miasmen* unfortunately was not yet available at the time of going to press.

[19]   Quoted from Paschero [1959].

[20]   *Chronic Diseases* I, p. 151-153 of German original.

12

Comments on Hahnemann's Organon of Practical Medicine

The comments made in this chapter may provide the stimulus for source study and assist the reader to gain more rapid orientation in the use of this work. Cross-references are given to other paragraphs on the same subject.

The list of questions in section 6 provides an opportunity for critical assessment as to whether sufficient knowledge of homoeopathic therapy has been acquired.

Samuel Hahnemann has been given the last word. He enjoins us to be consistent in applying the principles of homoeopathy.

1 Source Studies as the Basis for Any Science

Three of the works which have come down to us from Samuel Hahnemann are of particular importance:

Materia Medica Pura

Chronic Diseases

The Organon of Practical Medicine

These books must be studied by everybody; someone else's discussion of them will not serve the purpose. If my own book has taught you anything it will now be obvious that source study and exegesis must lead to a deepening of knowledge and show us a way of successfully dealing with the problems our patients present to us in daily practice.

Source studies are not always easy, and I therefore offer some further assistance to help you save time in gaining a useful orientation on the *Organon*.

2 History of the *Organon*

1810   First edition appeared. Title: *Organon der rationellen Heikunde* (Organon of rational medical practice).

1819   2nd edition. Title changed to *Organon der Heilkunst* (Organon of practical medicine/medical practice).
        New maxim — *Aude sapere*

1824   3rd edition
1829   4th edition
1833   5th edition
1841-42 Revision (written by hand) for 6th edition. Hahnemann was then in his 86th year, and the new edition appeared posthumously. His wife Melanie delayed publication after his death.
1920   Richard Haehl acquired the complete literary estate from the Boenninghausen family who were subsequent heirs; this included the handwritten revision.
1921   6th edition published by Richard Haehl.

3 A Book Read All Over the World

The *Organon* has been translated into all major languages and has reached all corners of the earth. In 1979, an exhibition on the *Organon* was put on in Hamburg which was given the title 'Ein Buch geht um die Welt'[1] There must be something special about this book. It is up to us to make this work we have inherited one of real value to ourselves and our patients. Its significance can be grasped at the level of the mind but also in our hearts.

The *Organon* is a workbook, a guide to the practice of homoeopathic medicine. The quality of this work bases on Hahnemann's skill of accurate observation, and it can be used more or less as it stands. As far as his theoretical views are concerned, much has to be critically assessed today, for these belonged to another age. Yet there is also much which may be perceived to be the work of a man of vision, though we cannot yet penetrate it with the intellect.

Many find the original difficult to read. Our language and terminology has changed. Hochstetter has produced a new edition which is faithful to the content but uses more modern language. My personal preference is for the original.

> Even the best of copies will never be completely equal to the original. It lacks the originality, the artist's individual touch which is revealed in the work itself and determines the impression to be gained from it. The same applies to the *Organon*. We will only gain real understanding of Hahnemann's work if we follow the exposition of his ideas with careful attention. (Lorbacher)[2]

Of course, long convoluted sentences with numerous footnotes and comments are not to everybody's taste, for the line of argument is constantly broken. My advice to you is to read every paragraph twice, first without footnotes and comments and then as a whole.

4 General Design of the Book

The *Organon* begins with a Preface and an Introduction. The Prefactory Memorandum from the 1810 edition is also included.

Preface A discussion of the therapy and radical measures used in contemporary medicine; the advantages of Hahnemann's own approach are shown up in contrast to these, and the reader is enjoined to keep homoeopathy pure.

Introduction Hahnemann discusses the disadvantages of the old method in detail, with particular reference to the underlying idea that disease is something tangible, something to be got rid of (*materia peccans*). This explains the radical derivative therapies used (venesection, emetics, purges, laxatives). In contrast to this, his own concept of disease is that of a dynamic imbalance, with the harmony of the vital energies disrupted. The vital energies maintain life in a state of health. If there is imbalance, they lose their capacity for self-regulation and healing has to be initiated from without, through the drug. Drug diagnosis according to the Law of Similars. Classic formulation of the Law of Similars: 'To achieve a gentle, rapid, certain and lasting cure, always choose a drug capable of provoking a disease similar (*homoion pathos*) to the one it is to cure.'

The text proper is divided into paragraphs, with three main sections:

1 Theoretical basis (§§ 1-70)
2 Application in practice (§§ 71-285)
3 Adjuvant measures (§§ 286-291)

The text shows a clear logical structure. This is more easily discernible if it is realized that major topics are presented from three angles — first presenting the problem, then theoretical discussion and substantiation, and finally the practical consequences.

The synopsis given below provides cross-references to paragraphs relating to the same topics (third column).

5 Synopsis

Main topic	*Contents*	*Cross-references*
	I Theoretical Basis (§§ 1-70)	
The physician's role/1-2	Effect a cure rather than theorize Cure must be rapid, gentle, lasting	Introduction 'To achieve a gentle . . .
Synopsis and composition of the work:	The physician must be well informed concerning:	

III Adjuvant Measures (§§ 286-291)

Baths and massage may be given during convalescence once the basic disease has been cured. As Kneipp was to do later, Hahnemann recommended cold water applications, particulary if vital warmth was lacking.   291

6 List of Questions

Section 3 succinctly states the basic knowledge required for the effective practice of homoeopathic medicine. At a quiet moment the reader may now test himself, having reached the end of this book.

Definition of disease	Imbalance in the self-governing vital energies (§ 11)
How is the disease recognized?	On the basis of the totality of symptoms (§ 7)
How do we obtain the symptoms?	By taking a careful, individualized case history (§§ 84, 104)
Which are the important symptoms?	Remarkable, peculiar, unusual and singular (characteristic) symptoms (§ 153)
How is drug action defined?	It produces morbid symptoms in healthy subjects (§ 21) — a form of artificial disease (§ 34)
How are drug actions determined?	In drug tests on healthy subjects (§ 108)
How do the drugs effect a cure?	The drug-induced disease is stronger than the natural disease (§ 26)
How should the drug-induced disease relate to the natural disease?	They should be similar in symptomatology (§ 25). The classic formulation is given in the Introduction (cf. Chapter 2, p. 21)
How are the drugs prepared?	By potentization (§ 269)
Which potency should be used?	The one most appropriate to overcome the natural disease (§§ 275, 279)
At what intervals are drugs repeated?	More frequently in acute illnesses, though dissolved in water and succussed; in chronic illness less frequently and in higher potencies, or daily in LM potencies (§§ 246, 248, 270)
Finally the crucial question: 'What are your views on compound drugs?'	'It is wrong to use complex means where simple means will do.' (§§ 273, 274)

7 The Final Word is Samuel Hahnemann's

'Homoeopathy thus is a very simple form of medical practice, consistent in its principles and methods. Like the theory on which it is based it may be seen to be . . . complete in itself and therefore effective on its own. Integrity in theory and practice should be a matter of course, with no return whatsoever . . . to wrong ways if pride is to be taken in the reputable name of 'homoeopathy'.[3]

[1] 'A book read all over the world'. The exhibition was initiated by Schweitzer who also published a book with the same title.
[2] Cf. *Organon* 6th edn, Editor's Preface to the German edn publ. by Haug.
[3] Preface to the 6th edn of the *Organon*.

INDEX OF LITERATURE

Allen, Henry C.: Keynotes and Characteristics. New Delhi 1979 (reprint)
____: Materia Medica of the Nosodes. New Delhi 1977 (reprint)
Allen, John Henry: The Chronic Miasms. Bombay 1969 (reprint)
Allen, Timothy F.: The Encyclopedia of pure Materia Medica. New Delhi 1976 (reprint)
Balzer, B. u. *Rolli, S.*: Sozialtherapie mit Eltern Behinderter. Beltz, Weinheim u. Basel 1975
Bamm, Peter: Ex Ovo, Essays über die Medizin, Stuttgart 1956
Barthel, Horst/Klunker, Will: Synthetisches Repertorium, 3 Bände. Heidelberg 1974
Baumann, U. (ed): Indikation zur Psychotherapie. Urban & Schwarzenberg, München-Wien-Baltimore 1981
Baur, J./Schweitzer, W.: Ein Buch geht um die Welt. Heidelberg 1979
Bayr, Georg: Kybernetik und homöopathische Medizin. Heidelberg 1969
Becker, H.: Konzentrative Bewegungstherapie. Thieme, Stuttgart 1981
Berger, M.: Der Patient ist auch ein Mensch. Hippokrates, Stuttgart 1981
Beuchelt, Hellmuth: Homöopathische Konstitutionstypen. Ulm/Donau 1956
____: Homöopathische Reaktionstypen. Ulm/Donau 1960, 3. Aufl.
Bidwell, Glen Irving: How To Use The Repertory with A Practical Analysis of Forty Homeopathic Remedies. Saffron Walden: Health Science Press, n.d.
Bier, August: Homöopathie und harmonische Ordnung der Heilkunde. Harausgegeben von Dr. Oswald Schlegel. Stuttgart 1949, 2. Aufl.
Boenninghausen's Therapeutic Pocket Book. Herausgegeben von Timothy Field Allen. New Delhi o. J. (reprint)
Boericke, William: Pocket Manual of Homoeopathic Materia Medica. B. Jain, New Delhi 1984 (reprint).
Borland, Douglas M.: Children's Types. The British Hom. Association, London

Bowen, M.: Family therapy in clinical practice. Aronson, New York 1978

Braun Artur: Methodik der Homöotherapie. Regensburg 1975

Burton, G.: Praktische Psychologie für Krankenpflegeberufe. Urban &
Schwarzenberg, München-Wien 1977

Charette, Gilbert: Homöopathische Arzneimittellehre für die Praxis.
Übersetzung Dr. Stockebrand. Stuttgart, 2. Aufl., 1978

Clarke, John H.: Hahnemann and Paracelsus. London 1923

Curry, Manfred: Der Schlüssel zum Leben. Zürich 1935

Deichmann, H.: Die Lehre von den Hahnemann'schen Miasmen. in:
Zeitschrift für Klassische Homöopathie 1976, Heft 1

Dorcsi, Mathias: Symptomenverzeichnis. Ulm/Donau 1965

_____: Medizin der Person. Heidelberg 1980, 3. Aufl.

_____, Stufenplan und Ausbildungsprogramm in der Homöopathie.
Heidelberg 1980

Eichelberger, Otto: Klassische Homöopathie. Heidelberg 1979

_____: Fragebogen und Rundbrief zur Weiterbildung in klassischer
Homöopathie als Skriptum beim Verfasser

Eysenck, H. J.: Vererbung, Intelligenz und Erziehung, Stuttgart 1975

Ensinger, Th.: Leitfaden zu Kent's Repertorium. Heidelberg 1975

Faust, V. (ed): Der psychisch Kranke in unserer Gesellschaft. Hippokrates,
Stuttgart 1981

Flury Rudolf: Praktisches Repertorium. Bern 1979 (Selbstverlag).

_____: Realitätserkenntnis und Homöopathie. Herausgeber Dr. med.
Gerhard Resch und Mechtild Flury-Lemberg. Engl. edition: Dr Flury's
Practical Repertory. Homoeopathy and the Principle of Reality. Trs.
Meuss. Berne: M. Flury-Lemberg 1979

Foubister, D. M.: Homöopathische Anamneseerhebung bei Kindern.
In: Zeitschrift für klassische Homöopathie. VI/2 Ulm/Donau 1962

Fritsche, Herbert: Samuel Hahnemann, Idee und Wirklichkeit der
Homöopathie. Stuttgart 1954

Gastpar, A.: Die Behandlung Geisteskranker. Enke, Stuttgart 1902

Gebser, Jean: Ursprung und Gegenwart. Stuttgart 1966, 2. Aufl.

Gebhardt, K. H. (Hrsg.): Beweisbare Homöopathie. Heidelberg 1980

Gnaiger, Jutta: Der geschwätzige Mensch. In: Allgemeine
Homöopathische Zeitung, Bd. 223/6. Heidelberg 1978

Goetze, H.: Personenzentrierte Spieltherapie. Hogrefe, Göttingen 1980

Haehl, Richard: Samuel Hahnemann, His Life and Work. Trs. Wheeler
/Grundy, ed. Clarke/Wheeler. London: Hom. Publ. Co. 1922

Hahnemann Samuel: The Organon of Medicine. Most recent translation
by Kunzli/Naude/Pendleton. London: Victor Gollancz 1983

_____: Materia medica pura. 2 vols. Trs. Dudgeon. New Delhi: B. Jain
1983 (reprint)

_____: The Chronic Diseases, Their Peculiar Nature and Their Homeopathic Cure. 2 vols. Trs. L. Tafel, ed. Pemberton, annot. R. Hughes. New Delhi: B. Jain 1981 (reprint)

Hering, Carl: The Guiding Symptoms of our Materia Medica. New Delhi 1974 (reprint)

Hochstetter, Kurt: Einführung in die Homöopathie. Regensburg 1973. Organon der Heilkunst. Neue Überarbeitung des Werkes von Samuel Hahnemann. Regensburg 1978

Homöopathisches Arzneibuch: 3. Aufl. 1978

Huter, Carl: Menschenkenntnis durch Körperformen- und Gesichtsausdruckskunde. Schwaig b/Nürnberg 1957. 3. Aufl.

Ide, Dr.: Die Zeiten des Auftretens und der Verschlimmerung der Beschwerden mit ihren vorzüglichen Arzneien. Sonderdruck, Herkunft nicht feststellbar. (Ausleihe: Homöopathische Bibliothek, Hamburg)

Imhäuser, Hedwig: Homöopathie in der Kinderheilkunde. Heidelberg 1970

Itschner, Viktor (Hrsg.): Potenzierte Heilmittel. Stuttgart 1971

Jahr, G. H. G.: Allgemeine und spezielle Therapie der Geisteskrankheiten und Seelenstörungen nach homöopathischen Grundsätzen, Leipzig 1855

Jonas, A. D.: Kurzpsychotherapie in der Allgemeinmedizin. Hippokrates, Stuttgart 1981

Julian, O.: Materia Medica der Nosoden. Heidelberg 1975. 2. Aufl.

Kästner, Erhard: Aufstand der Dinge. Frankfurt/Main 1973

Kaufmann, L.: Familie, Kommunikation, Psychose. Huber, Bern-Stuttgart 1972

Keller, Georg von: Kent's Repertorium. Neu übersetzt und herausgegeben. Ulm/Donau 1960

_____: Symptomensammlung homöopathischer Arzneimittel. Heidelberg 1972-79

Kent, J. T.: Final General Repertory of the Homoeopathic Materia Medica. Revised and augmented by Pierre Schmidt and Diwan Harish Chand. New Delhi: National Homoeopathic Pharmacy 1982.

_____: Repertory of the Homoeopathic Materia Medica. New Delhi: World Homoeopathic Links 1982 (reprint)

_____: Lectures on Homoeopathic Philosophy. New Delhi: B. Jain 1983 (reprint)

_____: What the Doctor Needs to Know in Order to Make a Successful Prescription. New Delhi: B. Jain 1980 (reprint)

Kindt, H.: Der Umgang mit psychisch Kranken. Kohlhammer, Stuttgart 1980

Klunker W.: Synthetic Repertory. Vol. 3: Sleep Dreams and Sexuality. Heidelberg: Haug 1974

Köhler, Gerhard: Über die Modalität Zeit. In: Deutsche Homöopathische Monatsschrift, 1958/12. Stuttgart 1958

____: Die Zeiten der Arznei. In: Erfahrungsheilkunde IX/1. Ulm/Donau 1960

____: Eine bildhafte Studie über das Symptom >Angst<. In: Deutsche Homöopathische Monatsschrift, 7 (1960)

____: Homöopathie. In: Wörterbuch medizinischer Grundbegriffe. Herausgegeben von Eduard Seidler, Freiburg 1979

____: Skripten über verschiedene Krankheitssyndrome und ihre homöopathische Behandlung. (Beim Verfasser anzufordern)

Korsakoff, von: Erfahrungen über ein völlig sicheres und leichtes Verfahren, die homöopathischen Arzneien zu jedem beliebigen Grade potenzieren zu können. In: Stapfs Archiv. 11 (1832)

Kretchmer, E.: Körperbau und Charakter. Berlin 1936

Künzli v. Fimelsberg, Jost: Kent's Repertorium. Neu übersetzt und herausgegeben (siehe von Keller) Ulm/Donau 1960

____: Hahnemanns Repertorien. In: Acta Homöopathica XIII/1. Heidelberg 1969

Ledermann, E.K.: Homoeopathy and the existential-phenomenological approach. Br Hom J 1966; 55:4

Leers, Hans: Sammlung seltener Symptome. Heidelberg 1973

____: Kents Repertorium in Lochkartenform. Solingen 1979, 4. Aufl.

Leeser, O.: Textbook of Homoeopathy. 6 vols. Heidelberg: Haug n.d.

Leibbrand, Werner: Romantische Medizin. Hamburg 1937

Martini, Paul: Homöopathische Arzneimittel-Nachprüfungen. In: Naunyn-Schmiedebergs Archiv für experimentelle Pathologie und Pharmakologie. Bd. 192, Bonn 1939

Mezger, Julius: Gesichtete homöopathische Arzneimittellehre. Saulgau 1951

Müller, H. V.: Das Krankheitsgeschehen aus homöopathischer Sicht. In: Zeitschrift für Klassische Homöopathie 1978, Heft 1

Nash, E.B.: Leaders in Homoeopathic Therapeutics. New Delhi: B. Jain 1983 (reprint)

Pandy, K.: Irrenfürsorge in Europa. Reimer, Berlin 1908

Paschero, Tomas Pablo: Die homöopathische Diagnose. In: Zeitschrift für klassische Homöopathie. III/6. Ulm/Donau 1959

____: Diagnosis of the similimum. Br Hom J 1964; 53:88.

____: Homöopathie als konstitutionelle Medizin. In: Zeitschrift für klassische Homöopathie. VI/2. Ulm/Donau 1962

Pavel, F. G.: Die klientenzentrierte Psychotherapie, Pfeiffer, München 1978

Petzold, H. (ed): Dramatische Therapie. Hippokrates, Stuttgart 1981

Redlich, F. C./Freedman, D. X.: Theorie und Praxis der Psychiatrie. (Übertragen aus dem Amerikanischen) Frankfurt/Main 1974, 2. Aufl.

Remschmidt, H.: Psychologie für Krankenpflegeberufe. 2. Aufl. Thieme, Stuttgart 1977

Ritter, Hans: Samuel Hahnemann. Sein Leben und Werk in neuer Sicht. Heidelberg 1974

Roberts, Herbert A.: Sensations as if —. A Repertory of Subjective Symptoms. New Delhi 1983 (reprint)

Schlüren, Erwin: Homöopathie in Frauenheilkunde und Geburtshilfe. Heidelberg 1977

Schmeer, D. H.: Die Differentialdiagnose neurotischer und homöopathischer Symptome. In: Zeitschrift für klassische Homöopathie. XII/6 (1968)

_____: Die homöopathische Behandlung der Neurosen. In: Acta Homöopathica. XIII/4 (1969)

Schneider, W.: Der schwierige Patient. Hoffmann-La Roche, Grenzach 1978

Schoeler, Heinz:Über die wissenschaftlichen Grundlagen der Homöopathie. Über angewandte Toxikologie. Leipzig 1948 (reprint DHU Karlsruhe 1978)

Schraml, W. J.: Psychologie im Krankenhaus. 3. Aufl. Huber, Bern-Stuttgart-Wien 1975

Schultz, Carl Heinrich: Die homöobiotische Medizin des Theophrastus Paracelsus. Berlin 1831

Schulz, Hugo: Vorlesungen über Wirkung und Anwendung der unorganischen Arzneistoffe. Ulm/Donau 1956 (reprint)

_____: Vorlesungen über Wirkung und Anwendung der deutschen Arzneipflanzen. Ulm/Donau 1956 (reprint)

Schweitzer, Wolfgang: Ein Buch geht um die Welt, Heidelberg 1979

Seidler, Eduard: Geschichte der Pflege des kranken Menschen. Stuttgart 1972

_____: Wörterbuch medizinischer Grundbegriffe. Freiburg 1979

Speight, Phyllis: A comparison of the Chronic Miasms, Rustington/Sussex 1961

Stauffer, Carl: Homöotherapie. Regensburg 1924

_____: Symptomenverzeichnis. Regensburg 1951, 3. Aufl.

Stiefvater, Erich: Akupunktur als Neuraltherapie. Ulm/Donau 1956, 2. Aufl.

Tischner, Rudolf: Samuel Hahnemann. Leben und Lehre. Ulm/Donau 1959

____: Geschichte der Homöopathie, 4 Bände, Leipzig 1934

____: Das Werden der Homöopathie, Stuttgart 1950

Tompkins, Peter und *Bird, Christopher*. Das geheime Leben der Pflanzen. Frankfurt/ M. 1978

Tyler, M.: A study of Kent's Repertory. Br Hom J 1983; 72:130 (reprinted)

Tyler M & Weir J.: Repertorizing. Br Hom J 1983; 72:195 (reprinted)

____: Uses of the Repertory and 'Repertorizing'. New Delhi: B. Jain n.d. (reprint)

Vehhsemeier, Albert: In: Hygea, 4. Band, Karlsruhe 1836

Voegeli, Adolf: Die rheumatischen Erkrankungen. Ulm/Donau 1961

Voisin, Henri: Die vernünftige kritische Anwendung der Homöopathie. Übersetzt und herausgegeben von Dr. med. Fritz Stockebrand. Ulm/Donau 1960

____: Materia Medica des homöopathischen Praktikers. Übersetzung von Dr. Heinrich Gerd-Witte. Heidelberg 1969

____: Praktische Homöotherapie. Übersetzt, verlegt und herausgegeben von Dr. F. und P. Stockebrand. Hamm 1969

Vonessen, Franz: 'Was krank macht, ist auch heilsam'. Heidelberg 1980

Wachsmuth, Guenther: Erde und Mensch. Konstanz 1952, 2. Aufl.

Ward, James William: Unabridged Dictionary of the Sensations 'As if'. New Delhi 1983 (reprint)

Weiss, R. F.: Lehrbuch der Phytotherapie. Stuttgart 1979, 4. Aufl. English edition of this authoritative work on herbal medicine due to appear shortly.

Weizsäcker, Viktor v.: Studien zur Pathogenese. Leipzig 1935

Wolter, Hans: Wirksamkeitsnachweis von Caulophyllum D 30 bei der Wehenschwäche des Schweines. Die Wirksamkeit von Flor de Piedra D 3 bei der Azetonämie des Rindviehs. In: Beiweisbare Homöopathie. (Siehe Gebhardt) Heidelberg 1980

Wurmser, Lise: Die Entwicklung der homöopathischen Forschung, Karlsruhe o. J. (Sonderdruck DHU)

INDEX